# Spell Craft Primer

A guide to understanding the basics of spell workings

Library of Congress -in-Publication Data
September 2011

The instructions, descriptions, and recipes in this book are provided for entertainment purposes only.

Individual reactions to the contained materials can vary.  It is not possible to predict how any individual or area of your home will react to a particular recipe, treatment, or ingredient.

As with any product common sense should be used when creating these recipes, following these instructions, or attempting any ritual included within this guide.

The enclosed materials are for informational purposes only and the reader accepts all responsibility for determining the effectiveness and usefulness of all included information.  Neither the author nor the publisher accepts and liability for the actions of the reader nor for any reactions caused by the use of the contents and ingredients.

To obtain information or inquire about availability please write to Director, PO Box 1, Hollidaysburg, PA 16648

# Spell Craft Primer

A guide to understanding the basics of spell workings

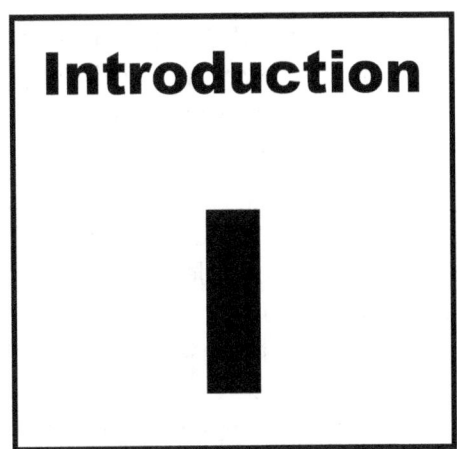

# Introduction

**I**

Alternative therapy comes in many forms. Some people believe strongly in the benefits of aromatherapy while others believe only in the benefits of herbs, oils, and extracts. Some people think that the natural world can only be employed to exert a positive effect by spell casting while others see holistic medical practitioners as a means to achieve physical and emotional well-being.

As you expand your understanding of the methods employed in alternative therapy, you will see many instances where science and spell casting overlap. Each therapy employs similar energy channeling, herbs, oils, extracts, or methodology to achieve the same benefit.

The purpose of this particular book is to illustrate some of the most commonly used elements in spell casting and to give you a bit of insight into how these elements transcend the barrier between spell casting and science.

- ➤ Acupuncture is a traditional health treatment that uses needles to stimulate energy points within the body to help treat conditions ranging from the physical to the emotional.

- ➤ Acupressure and stimuli massages rely on pressure points within the body to stimulate ki or chi energy points that promote the release of energies and open blockages within the body's energy flow.

- ➤ Aromatherapy is the use of scent to help improve a person's health and well-being. Aromatherapy relies on massage, inhalations, baths, diffusers, or vaporizers to release beneficial aromas into the air.

- ➤ Ayurvedic Medicine is a system of medicine that treats the whole. It incorporates a variety of methodology including detoxification, diet, exercise, herbology, and stimuli to improve emotional, mental, and physical heath.

- ➤ Chiropractic care is the belief that the health and movement of the musculoskeletal system affects every aspect of the human body. Manipulation of the musculoskeletal system is believed to alleviate or prevent ailments within every body system.

- ➤ Color therapy relies on the concept that every color operates on its own frequency. The body contains energy. This energy also has a frequency. Using the energy frequencies of color, therapists adjust the imbalances in the frequency of the body's energy to a healthy level.

- ➤ Crystal & Gemstone therapy also relies on energy frequencies. Each crystal and gemstone has a definite atomic structure. The structure of each crystal enables it to release specific energy. This energy is then channeled to aid the body in balancing its own energy.

- ➤ Herbalism is the practice of using plants and herbs to treat or prevent physical and emotional ailments. These practices rely on the chemical components found in the herb and the ability of these chemicals to affect the body.

- ➤ Homeopathy is a form of holistic medicine that uses animal, vegetable, and mineral components to cure an illness.

- ➤ Hypnotherapy & psychic trances are methods employed to focus the powers of the mind and facilitate the minds abilities.

- ➤ Meditation, relaxation, and visualization are all methods of calming the mind & body and focusing energies while using positive visualization to overcome mental, emotional, and physical barriers.

- ➤ Nutritional Therapy is a form of preventative medicine that relies on the incorporation of a special diet into a healthy lifestyle to balance the body and prevent illness. Some therapists make adjustments to the diet to aid the body in healing from a particular ailment.

➤ Polar therapy is a balancing of the energies in the body to achieve health for both the mind and the body. The concept of polar therapy relies on the understanding that the body is like a living magnet where energy flows between positive and negative poles. When the energy within the body flows freely between poles, the body & mind are aligned.

➤ Reflexology is the science of applying pressure to the feet and hands to stimulate a reactive response in a related muscle, organ system, or energy within the body.

➤ Spiritual healing is the use of the energy that flows around the mind, body, and spirit to keep the person as a whole in working order. When these energies become damaged, the natural healing mechanisms in the body become inadequate. Spiritual healing relies on a conductor to channel healing energy where ever it is needed to mend this flow of energy around the body.

Spell craft related to physical and emotional health is an approach that blends many of these therapies into one working set of treatments. The ritual of spell craft comes in many, many forms. Spell craft pre-dates many of the other methodologies currently being employed to treat the mind, body, and spirit.

The purpose of this guide is to give you a fundamental understanding of spell craft as well as some starter instructions to enable you to begin on your path to channeling the energies around you to benefit yourself and those who come to you for aide. Each section is defined for you in a way that enables you to begin on the path to understanding the power you hold within you and the methods you can employ to channel that power and the power of the world.

If you find a section that works well with your personal powers and energies, we encourage you to pursue additional knowledge and learning. Every element affects every other element. For example, we provide a basic description of the benefits of each phase of the moon in relationship to general spell work. If moon magic is of particular interest to you, you should pursue enhanced learning regarding the power of each phase of the moon.

You will notice that instructions employ many of the other alternative healthcare methodologies. Modern science is illustrating to alternative healthcare practitioners what generations of spell casters already knew. The energy in the world can be channeled to effect a positive change in the mind, body, and spirit.

The recipe sections of the guide operates under the understanding gained through generations of practitioners backed up by modern scientific research into the properties of certain stones, metals, herbs, oils, and extracts. These inclusions are designed for general use but each person varies from the next. You may wish to obtain a **Compendium of Beneficial Herb & Oils** similar to the one I have available to aid you in selecting the proper ingredients for the results you desire.

Most people think of spells as a process that they need to follow to cast the spell and they envision the instructions as a recipe. Many of the inclusions in this guide do follow the form of a recipe giving you ingredients and steps to follow. Following the instructions is important, but equally important is the intent and will of the person following each 'recipe'.

Equal in importance to the instructions with each recipe is your intent. You must have a clear goal in mind while you complete each step in the process. Your goal should be a benefit that you can visualize and focus on while you complete each step.

If the instructions in this guide are not providing the benefit you desire, you might wish to take some contemplation time before making another attempt.

Each of these 'recipes' can only work with the energies of the world and according to the rules of nature.

A weight loss cure will only work well if you aide the recipe by establishing healthy practices like restraint and exercise to support the beneficial effects of the ingredients and processes.

A love recipe or aphrodisiac will not work well if you doubt yourself or your partner.

Your personal self-confidence, intent, and supporting actions are as important to these recipes as the ingredients and instructions.

Luck is one example of a characteristic that some people are believed to have in abundance and that others attempt to attain through spell casting. We have all heard someone say "They are so lucky" about another person. Luck, like anything, is dependent on many factors. You can help to channel the natural world to increase your luck, but you must also believe in yourself and your ability to BE lucky.

Belief in self is the first, and most important, ingredient in good luck work. In fact, belief in your ability to channel the natural world to achieve your goals is the most important ingredient to success in any endeavor.

Belief is your first and most important tool.

There are many other tools that you will use to aid your natural abilities. Some are used repeatedly because they have certain properties, uses, and associations. These are called correspondences. Each section will have a general correspondence chart to illustrate to you how others employ the "ingredients" but you must gain inner knowledge to determine the correct correspondences for your personal energy.

**CHAPTER 1**

## Centering, Grounding, & Shielding

The act of grounding and centering is meant to give you a stable foundation for shielding yourself and channeling the energy in yourself and the world around you.

The mind and the body function as one unit. The mind and body contain energy frequencies that interact with the world around us.

1.    Find a position that is relaxing for you.

2.    Tense and relax every part of your body beginning at the feet and moving to your head visualizing all of your tension leaving each part.

    ➤    Start with the toes.

    ➤    Tense your toes.  Hold the tension for 10 seconds.

    ➤    Relax your toes releasing all of the stress and worry contained within your toes.

    ➤    Move to your feet.

3.    Breathe slowly and evenly during the relaxation process.

    ➤    Inhale as you tense each part of your body
    ➤    Exhale as you release that tension.

4.    Feel each part of your body relax and loose all of the world's tension.

> Expel the tension with each breath you take.

5.    When you are completely relaxed, visualize a place that is beautiful and calming to you.

6.    Focus all of your senses on that place.

My place is a forest.

> Feel the place as well or better than you feel your true environment

I can feel the light moisture in the air, the softness of the pine needles underneath my body, and warmth of the sunlight filtering through the tall tress.

> See the details of the place that you have chosen

I can see the beauty of the sunlight reflecting off the trees, the wind filtering through the leaves and groundcover and the forest animals going about the business of life

> Smell the air

I can smell the fresh clean sent of new growth and the warm, comforting smell of old leaves, branches, and other matter returning to the soil.

> Hear the sounds

I can hear the wind rustling the trees and the sounds that the birds and animals make as they forage for food or play in the trees.

7.    When you have completely visualized the place that is relaxing and beautiful to you, make yourself a part of that place.

> Feel your body become one with the place you have chosen.

I feel my body become one with the most beautiful tree in the forest planted solidly in the earth.

I feel my roots dig deep beneath the surface keeping me solidly within my favorite place planting me solidly in the world.

8. Ground yourself within your favorite place and take the energy that the place has to offer into yourself.

I feel my roots gaining the sustenance of all that has lived in the forest before.

I feel my branches reach toward the sunlight gathering the warmth and energy of the sun.

9. Feel your strength.

I feel myself planted firmly within the forest, a vital and giving part of my favorite place while I gain strength from the world.

10. When you are ready, open your eyes, and return to the world around you knowing that you are well grounded and carry the strength of the world within your body.

As you become more adept at relaxation and visualization, you will be able to ground and center yourself more quickly and with fewer steps. You will also find that the feeling of relaxation, focus, and strength stay with you for longer periods of time.

# *Shielding*

Once you are relaxed, grounded, and energized by the world around you, you must shield yourself from the negative energies that may seek to break your focus or bring harm to your personal energies and sense of self. In spell craft this is known as shielding.

Always ground and center your mind and body before you attempt to shield yourself. Allowing negative energies to cling to you when you shield your mind and body can cause more harm than benefit.

1.   Complete the steps of relaxation and visualization.

2.   Before leaving your perfect place, picture all of your energy as a ball of light buried deep within the core of your body.

3.   Allow the ball of light to expand within your body, filling every part of you.

4.   When you can feel the ball of light reaching every part of your body from the top of your head to the ends of your toes, see it expand outside of your body like a bubble.

5.   Allow this bubble to draw the energy from deep within your core until you feel a strength surrounding every inch of your body expelling all negative energy as it surrounds you with strength.

6.   Seal the bubble to enclose every part of your body.

7.   Picture this impenetrable shield deflecting any negative energy that seeks to reach you.

As you become more adept at the processes necessary to ground, center, and shield, you will be able to shield yourself more quickly. It is important that you complete the steps to ground, center, and shield yourself every time you begin to feel weakened.

Certain talismans, stones, and crystals store protective energy. These aids help to strengthen you and create shields beyond what you can do with the energy of your mind & body alone.

You should scrutinize the sections relating to talismans, stones, and crystals to determine if you can benefit from the enhancements these can provide.

While there are many options that promote strength and protection, each of us has a slightly different frequency. You should select talismans, stones, and crystals that feel right to you because these are most likely to operate on the frequency you need to achieve the benefit you desire.

# Color Correspondences

You will select colors for each item you create. Many people believe in the power of color to influence our heath, emotions, and personal harmony.

Each color vibrates on its own frequency affecting the items around it. Each person is surrounded by an energy field called an aura. This energy field can become damaged or lose energy due to external or internal forces. The cells in your body also have an energy fields that operate on a specific frequency when you are healthy. When your body or mind loses that healthy frequency, color is believed to help restore the necessary harmony of the cells and help you to regain health.

Each type of therapy has a different method of using color. Color correspondences in spell work vary between practitioners as well.

The charts illustrate the most commonly used colors and their expected benefits. You should select the color that corresponds best with the goal of your spell or blend and that feels correct to you. As with any tool, the frequency of the vibrations must match the goal of the user but it must also match the frequency of the user. These colors are starting points, but you should select the one that feels right for you.

| Color | General |
|-------|---------|
| Blue | Healing; Protection; Money; Wisdom; Calm; Creativity; Patience; Astral Projection; Prophetic Dreams |
| Black | Crossing, Cursing, Money, Debauchery |
| Green | Drawing; Expanding; Money; Gambling; Nature; Luck; Fertility |
| | Finances; Physical Healing; Abundance; Growth |
| | Corresponds to the Heart Chakra |
| | Element Earth |
| | Dirty or muddy green corresponds to envy, hate, and sickness |
| Green & Black | Reversing Money Jinxes |
| Indigo | Help reduce phobias and stress |
| | Justice; Wisdom; Inspiration; Intuition; Spirituality; Psychic Powers |
| Light or True Blue | Peace; Healing; Tranquility; Patience; Health |
| Orange | Communications; Opens Doors; Change; Happiness; Excitement; Assertiveness; Motivation, Persistence, Prosperity; Procrastination; Anxiety; Stress |
| | Solutions or new ways of accomplishing your goals. |
| | Corresponds to Navel |
| Pink | Love; Nurturing; Tenderness; Sensitivity; Harmony; Femininity; Innocence; Friendship; Drawing; Attraction; Morality; Honor; Romantic Peace; Nurturing |

| Purple | Artistic |
| --- | --- |
| | Creativity; Mastery; Commanding; Psychic Power; Inspiration; Spirituality; Intuition; Imagination; Royalty; Wealth; Inner Peace; Security; Protection; Business Progress; Ambition; Success; Independence |
| | Corresponds to The Crown Chakra |
| Red | Protection; Conflict; War; Passion; Sex; Strengthen Body; Love, Health; Energy; Passion; Career Goals; Courage |
| | Red corresponds to the Element fire |
| Red & Black | Reversing Spells |
| | Reversing Love Jinxes |
| Silver | Emotional Healing; Nurturing; Calming; Feminine Energy;, Balance; Harmony; Change; Learning; Introspection; Confidence; Wealth, Secrets; Hidden Desires; Intuition; Telepathy; Clairvoyance; Dreams; Astral Energy |
| | Corresponds to the Moon |
| White | Emotional Healing; Nurturing; Calming; Fertility; Blessing; Truth; Purity; Peace; Spirituality; Higher Self; Consecration; Divination; Clairvoyance |
| | White carries the powers of all the colors |
| Yellow | Success; Achievement; Goals, Purification; Money (gold); Gambling; Luck; Cheerfulness; Intellect; Hope; Direction; Personal Power; Clear Thinking; Concentration; Communication; Confidence; Persuasion; Learning; Breaking Mental Blocks |
| | It can also correspond to fear and treachery |
| | Corresponds to The Solar Plexus Chakra |
| | Bright yellows tend to carry the positive aspects, while pale or muddy yellows tend to carry the negative |

**CHAPTER 3**

## Candle Correspondences

One of the most common methods of natural magic and aromatherapy is candle burning. Most of us have used candles in our lives to scent a room, relax, or create a specific atmosphere.

Practitioners use candles in much the same way. The size and shape of the candle is not important. The colors of the candles are used in much the same way as color therapy. The difference is that therapeutic candles are infused with herbs & oils whose benefits have been proven through generations of use and often, by modern scientific research.

| Color | General Belief |
|-------|----------------|
| Blue | Create Confidence, Discover Truth, Expand Mental Horizons, Success, Protection, Good Fortune, Opening Blocked communication, Wisdom, Protection, Spiritual Inspiration, Calm, Reassurance |
| Black | Banishing, Leaving a Relationship, Acknowledging Grief, Forgiveness, Protection Repelling Negativity, Binding |
| Brown | Locating Lost Objects, Home Protection, Pet Protection, Money, Ideas, Balance, Influence Friendships, Special Favors |
| Copper | Passion, Money Goals, Professional Growth, Fertility in Business, Career Maneuvers |

| Gold | Worldly Achievement, Wealth, Recognition, Long Life, Winning |
|---|---|
| Green | Healing, Gardening, Tree Magic, Growth, Good Harvest, Prosperity, Money, Good Luck, Abundance, Fertility |
| Orange | Business Goals, Property Deals, Ambition, Career Goals, General Success, Justice, Legal Matters, Selling, Action |
| Pink | Love, Romance, Friendship, Affection, Quiet Sleep, Rekindling Trust, Attracting New Friends or Lovers, Healing Emotions, Peace |
| Purple | Meditation, Past-Life Work, Divination, Astral Travel, Psychic Protection, Nightmare Prevention, Remembrance for Parted Loved Ones, Influencing People, Spiritual Power, Self Assurance |
| Red | Courage, Energy, Strength, Career Goals, Fast Action, Lust, Vibrancy, Driving Force, Love, Survival Determination, Sexual Passion, Potency, Physical Health, Willpower |
| Silver | Divination, Astral Projection, Intuition |
| White | Protection, Cleansing, Divination, Healing, Clear Vision |
| Yellow | Mental Acumen, Gaining Approval, Improves Memory, Increase Concentration, Sharpen Logic, Intelligence |

You should always a new candle for each ritual you complete. Some people prefer to make their own candles for each particular use while others prefer to purchase ready made candles from another practitioner or a mass market store.

When you are finished with a candle, do not blow or pinch the flame away. This may have the effect of blowing or snuffing out your desires. You should wave your hand gently over the flame to create enough air movement to put the candle out without dispersing the air more than necessary.

# *Simple Candle Making Instructions*

Specialty and craft stores sell candle making supplies including a variety of wax, wicks, molds, and colorants.

1.  Prepare your mold according to the instructions for the type of mold you are using.

2.  Thread the wick through the mold so that the end will stick out beyond the candle wax

3.  Heat the wax until it is a smooth liquid consistency

4.  Add oils, herbs, and colorants as desired

5.  Pour the heated wax & additives into the mold of your choice

6.  Allow the wax to cool and harden

7.  Remove the finished candle from the mold if desired

8.  Some people prefer to infuse the candle with the necessary herbs & oils. Others prefer to dress the candle after it has been formed.

    You can rub the chosen oils into the candle wax beginning at the top and working downwards

9.  Use the preferred candle according to the beneficial remedy included in your preferred section

# Candle Magic

The benefits of colors, herbs, and oils have been proven through generations of use and through modern scientific research. You should use this understanding as a baseline for each spell you perform. You should also understand that the most effective spell would be the one that you create yourself using your thoughts, energies, and personal power.

Candles represent the element fire and make an excellent focus point for visualizing the results you desire. Lighting a charged candle may be sufficient for the goal you desire. Adding visualization and the ritual that seems the best to you will only serve to enhance the power of the candle.

1. Gather the tools that you need to complete the candle magic including

   ➢ the candle infused with the proper herbs & oils for your task

   ➢ any parchment or writing necessary for the task

   ➢ the spell you will use

   ➢ crystals, gemstones, talismans, or symbols you require

   ➢ symbolic representation of your goal or the person for whom you are completing the spell work

   ➢ any other item that you have incorporated into your spell plan

2. Complete the ritual preparation including centering, grounding, and shielding.

3. Visualize the goal you desire

4. Concentrate on what you want while completing the steps of your spell

5. Allow the candle to burn itself out or extinguish it according to your needs

**CHAPTER 4**

## Crystals and Gemstones

Crystals, like color, work at a specific energy level. Each crystal generates or stores a different energy. This energy radiates from the crystal in a way that can be beneficial to restoring the health of the energies in the body, mind, and soul.

Therapists in both traditional and non-traditional medicine use crystals to stimulate the body into self-healing, to restore the balance in the mind, and to channel the energy of the soul.

AGATE

Beneficial in stomach area

Restores energy and health

Good for transmutation.

Helps with the emotion of acceptance.

Brings happiness; emotional balance; wealth; health; and long life

AGATE / BOTSWANA

Eases stress; and pain of loss.

Reduces anxiety

AGATE / FIRE

Master healer with color therapy.

Enhances all essences

Grounds and balances

Sexual & heart chakra

Burns energy

AGATE / MOSS        Energizes colon; circulatory; pancreas; & pulses

Blood sugar balance

Emotional priorities; mental priorities

Aid in restoration of energy

Used in healing;

They are believed to bring the wearer happiness; wealth; health; and long life

Increases ability to ward off self-induced anger and inner bitterness

AGATE / PICTURE     L & R brain imbalances - epilepsy; autism; dyslexia; visual problems; blood circulation to the brain

Apathy is eased

ALEXANDRITE      Central nervous system disorders

Low self-esteem & difficulty centering

Stimulates happiness and pleasant surprises

Good fortune and success in speculative matters

AMBER          Thyroid; inner ear & neural-tissue strengthener

Memory loss; eccentric behavior; anxiety; inability to make decisions

Activates altruistic nature; realization of the spiritual intellect

Worn around the neck to help fight infection and respiratory diseases

Add strength to spells

Attract love; increase beauty

A Powerful healing stone which stores a large amount of cosmic and organic energy

| | |
|---|---|
| **AMETHYST** | Headaches; eyes; scalp; hair; pituitary gland; balancing blood sugar |
| | Amethyst is very effective as a healing stone |
| | Warmed and placed on the forehead and temples; it is good for headaches |
| | It is best worn near the heart center |
| | Psychic abilities; imagery |
| | Remove negativity |
| | Protection; increase intuition; helps to remember dreams |
| | Reduce anger; impatience; and nightmares |
| | Spiritually uplifting |
| | Spiritual awareness; peace; love; happiness; protection; divination and psychic work |
| **AQUAMARINE – LIGHT BLUE** | Heart; immune system; thymus; lymph nodes |
| | Calming; uplifting; flexibility; innocence; joy; creativity; communication; self-knowledge; confidence; purpose |
| | Releasing anxiety; fear; and restlessness |
| | Calms nervous tension |
| | It is most used to help banish fears and phobias |
| | A stone of joy and happiness |
| | Protective stone of the traveler |
| **APATITE** | Promotes communication and mental clarity |
| **AVENTURINE** | Eliminates psychosomatic ills; fear; skin diseases; nearsightedness |
| | Positive attitude; creative insight |
| | Increases mental powers; perception; and insight |
| | Considered the "Gamblers" stone |

| | |
|---|---|
| AZURITE | Arthritis & joints |
| | Helps one let go of old belief systems; dissolves fear & helps transform it into understanding |
| | Meditation; promoting psychic ability |
| AZURITE-MALACHITE | Skin diseases; anorexia; calms anxiety; lack of discipline |
| | Powerful healing force to physical body; emotional release |
| BERYL | Laziness; hiccoughs; swollen glands; eye diseases; bowel cancer |
| | Patience; humor; discipline |
| BLOODSTONE / HELIOTROPE | Circulation; all purpose healer & cleanser; stomach & bowel pain; purifies bloodstream; bladder; strengthens blood purifying organs |
| | Stimulates flow of energy for healing blood circulation; stops hemorrhaging |
| | Takes away negativity and sadness |
| | Removes emotional blockages |
| | Physical strength; courage; victory in court; exorcism |
| CALCITE | Healer and balancer of personal power |
| CARNELIAN | Circulatory system; kidneys; stimulate appetite; emotions; sexuality; physical energy; celebration; reproductive system; menstrual cramps; arthritis; kidneys; gall bladder; pancreas |
| | Eases depression; gives protection and energy |
| | A female stone; heals and balances the reproductive system |
| | Grounding; stimulates curiosity & initiative |
| CHALCEDONY | Fever; gallstones; leukemia; eye problems |
| | Touchiness; melancholy |
| | Stimulates maternal feelings & creativity |

CHRYSOCOLLA

Arthritis; feminine disorders; eases labor & birth

Emotional balance & comforter

Alleviates fear; guilt & nervous tension.

Facilitates clairvoyance

CHRYSOPGRASE

Gout; eye problems; promotes sexual organ strength

Alleviates greed; depression; hysteria & selfishness

CHRYSOLITE

Toxemia; viruses; appendicitis

Inspiration; prophecy

Prevents nightmares; increases psychic awareness

CITRINE

Acid indigestion; food disorders; allergies

Cleansing spleen; kidneys; liver; urinary system; intestines

It is an aid to the digestive system; and helps eliminate toxins

Mental and emotional clarity; problem-solving; memory; willpower; optimism; confidence; self-discipline

Reducing anxiety; fear; and depression

Encourages tremendous healing on the emotional and mental levels; helps unblock subconscious fears; and serves as a natural relaxant

Stimulates openness and accelerates the awakening of the mind

CITRINE QUARTZ

Heart; kidney; liver & muscle; appendicitis; gangrene; red & white corpuscles; digestive tract

Cleanses vibrations in the atmosphere

Creativity; helps personal clarity

Eliminates self-destructive tendencies

CORAL

Balances physical energy

Relaxes tension

22

Carries the creative vibrations of the sea

DIAMOND
Brain diseases; pituitary & pineal glands; draws out toxicity; poison remedy

Covers full spectrum of psychic and spiritual matters

DIOPSITE
Organ rejection

Heart; lung & kidney stimulation

Improves self-esteem

ELIAT STONE
Tissue & skeletal regeneration

Detoxifies

Antidepressant

Karmic life acceptance

EMERALD
Circulatory & neurological disorders

Respiratory system; heart; lymph nodes; blood; thymus; balance blood sugar; childbirth; eyesight

Lifts depression and insomnia

Increases psychic & clairvoyant abilities

Growth; peace; harmony; patience; love; monogamy; honesty

Promotes creativity

Stimulates perception and insight

Strengthens memory

EMERALD LIGHT
A stone of the heart

Beneficial effect on the eyes

Helps to clear emotional blockages; and understand life changes

FLOURITE
Bone disorders; anesthetic

Hyperkinesias; ability to concentrate; balances polarities; 3rd eye center; mental capacity & intellect

Reduce emotional involvement; gain perspective; increase mental power

Opens and softens the way for the use of other stones

| | |
|---|---|
| GARNET - RHODOLITE | Capillaries; skin elasticity; protection from pre- cancerous conditions |

GARNET - SPESSARTINE

Hormone imbalances; inflammations; sexual disease

Bad dreams; depression; anger; self esteem

GARNET

Light Pink to Deep Red

Strength; endurance; protection

Helps heals the eyes

Balancer of energies

Draws out negativity and bitterness

Helps elf-esteem; and encourages success in business

HEMATITE

Blood cleanser & purifier; self esteem; augments meridian flows; aids in astral projection

Stability; focus; and emotional balance

Calming to the emotions.

Worn as an amulet to confer strength and procure favorable legal judgments.

Used to reduce inflammation and treat hysteria.

Considered to be a grounding stone

Helps maintain balance between body; mind; and spirit

JADE

Heart; thymus; immune; kidney and cleansing blood; nervous system
Courage; knowledge; justice; compassion; emotional balance; humility; generosity; harmony; wealth; longevity
Stimulates practicality; wisdom; and universal attunement
Thought to provide a link between the spiritual and the mundane

JASPER - GREEN

Constipation; ulcers; intestinal spasms; bladder; gallbladder

Clairvoyance

For energy balancing of emotions and stress

| | |
|---|---|
| JASPER - PICTURE | Skin; kidneys; thymus & their neurological tissues; betters the immune system |
| | Past life recall |
| JASPER - RED | Liver; stomach troubles & infections |
| | Reduces stress and negativity |
| JASPER - YELLOW | Endocrine system tissue; thymus; pancreas; sympathetic ganglia stimulation |
| | Etheric body alignment |
| JET | Feminine disorders; teeth; stomach pain; glandular swelling; fevers; hair loss |
| KUNZITE | Alcoholism; anorexia; arthritis; epilepsy; gout; headaches; colitis; retardation; memory loss; schizophrenia & manic-depression |
| | Phobias; emotional equilibrium; self-esteem |
| KUNZITE - GREEN | Will heal pain from its originating point |
| KUNZITE - PINK | Will heal negative images of self; bringing peace |
| LAPIS | Neuralgia; melancholy; fevers; inflammations |
| | Focuses energy; public Speaking; spiritual cleanser; eliminates negative emotions |
| LAPIS - LAZULI | Dark blue with gold flecks helps to change negativity into positively |
| | Wisdom; truthfulness; psychic awareness; healing; strengthening when worn next to the skin |
| | Strengthens mind and body to spiritual awareness |
| LAZULITE | Frontal lobe stimulation; hypertension; liver diseases; immune system |

| MALACHITE | Draws out impurities on all levels; balances L & R brain functions; mental illness; co-ordination; vision |
| | All purpose healer; especially in solar plexus |
| | Money; protection; guards from danger |
| | Talisman to sleep soundly & protect from bad dreams |
| | Stimulates clear vision and insight; represents hope and inner peace |
| | Believed to protect from danger |
| | Increases abundance in all areas of life |
| MOONSTONE | Increases intuition |
| | Soothes & balances the emotions; helps eliminate emotional fear; encourages inner growth; aids peace |
| | Love; hope; protection; unselfishness; prophetic dreams |
| | Helps settle disputes |
| | Brings good fortune |
| | Reflects the wearers being and feelings |
| | Promotes unselfishness |
| | Good for protection while traveling on water |
| | Good for pre-menstrual symptoms and balancing to the reproductive system |
| | Used to ease childbirth |
| OBSIDIAN | Grounds and centers |
| | Protects from being abused; stabilizer; stomach; intestines; general muscle tissue healer; bacterial; viral inflammations |
| ONYX | Helps you to more forward |
| | Objective thinking; spiritual inspiration; control of emotions; help eliminate negative thinking; apathy; stress; neurological disorders |

| | |
|---|---|
| OPAL | Opens communications |
| | Spells involving children; protection; enhances intuition |
| OPAL - CHERRY | Blood disorders; depression; apathy; lethargy |
| | Intuition; joy |
| OPAL - DARK | Reproductive organs; spleen; pancreas |
| | Depression; balances; amplifies creative thought |
| OPAL - JELLY | Abdominal diseases |
| | Minimizes wide mood swings |
| | Mystical thought amplifier |
| OPAL - LIGHT | Balances L & R brain hemispheres for neural disorders; aids abdomen; pituitary; thymus problems |
| PEARL | Eliminates emotional imbalances; aids stomach; spleen; intestinal tract; ulcer problems |
| PERIDOT | Protects against nervousness; helps alleviate spiritual fear; aids in healing hurt feelings; instills physical vitality; amplifies other energies; creates positive emotional outlook; helps liver; adrenal function. |
| | Dispels fears; guilt; and depression |
| | Used to counteract negative emotions and healing of the spirit |
| | Affects top three chakras |
| PYRITE | Helps purify the bloodstream; upper respiratory tract; upper intestines; digestive aid; nervous exhaustion; grounding |
| QUARTZ - CLEAR | Amplifies healing energy |
| | Used to help draw out pain |
| | Protects from negative vibrations |

| QUARTZ - ROSE | Love, self-acceptance; emotional wounds; dissipates anger; tension; emotional balance; peacefulness; forgiveness; kindness; self-esteem |
|---|---|
| QUARTZ - YELLOW | Lymphatic cancer, circulatory problems |
| | Protection; mental awareness; improves visualization; helps focus attention; energy |
| QUARTZ - SMOKY | Hyperactivity; excess energy; grounding; depression; negative emotions; calming |
| RHODOCHROSITE | Narcolepsy;; poor eyesight |
| | Emotional trauma; mental breakdown; nightmares; hallucinations; forgiveness; protection; creative power; energy; love; peace |
| RHODONITE | Inner ear; anxiety; confusion; mental unrest |
| | Promotes calm; self worth; confidence; enhanced sensitivity |
| RHYOLITE | Balances emotions; self worth; enhances capacity to love; clarity |
| RUBY | Infections; cholesterol; blood clots; blood cleansing; impotency |
| | Self-esteem; love; courage; confidence; vitality; stamina; strength; leadership |
| | The stone of courage |
| RUTILE | Alleviates blockages within the psyche from childhood pressures |
| SAPPHIRE | Colic; rheumatism; mental illness; pituitary; anti- depressant; |
| | Spiritual enlightenment; inner peace; telepathy; clairvoyance; astral projection |
| SARDONYX | Mental self control; depression; anxiety; grief; meditation; wisdom; calming inner conflicts; soothes emotional states |

| | |
|---|---|
| SMITHSONITE | Eases fear of interpersonal relationships; merges astral & emotional bodies; balances perspective |
| SODOLITE | Oversensitivity; intellectual understanding; cleanses the mind. peace; meditation; wisdom; healing |
| SPINEL | Leg conditions; powerful general healer; detoxification aid |
| SUGILITE | Psychic powers; spirituality; healing wisdom |
| TIGER'S EYE | Focus; clears negativity; wealth; money; protection while traveling |
| TOPAZ | Balances emotions; calms passions; gout; blood disorders; hemorrhages; poor appetite; reverses aging; spiritual rejuvenation; endocrine system stimulation |
| | Releases tension; inspiration; soothing; calming; banishing nightmares; emotional balance; tranquility; restore physical energy |
| TOPAZ - BLUE | Helps clarity of thought and communication |
| TOPAZ - GOLD | Removes artistic blocks allowing creativity |
| TOPAZ  - WHITE | Helps to obtain material wants |
| TOURMELINE | Fear; negativity;  grief; calms nerves; concentration; genetic disorders; cancer; hormones; charisma; tranquil sleep. |
| | Causes the wearer to be more flexible; more understanding |
| TOURMELINE - BLACK | Arthritis; dyslexia; syphilis; heart diseases |
| | Anxiety; disorientation; raises altruism; deflects negativity; resentment; insecurity |
| TOURMELINE - BLUE | Lungs; larynx; thyroid; parasympathetic nerves |

| TOURMELINE - GREEN | Creativity; immune system; psychological problems; blood pressure; asthma |
| | Eliminates conflict within body & mind |
| TOURMELINE - RUBELLITE | Creativity; fertility |
| | Balances passive or aggressive nature |
| TOURMELINE - TURQUOISE | Heals; connects self to higher self |
| TURQUOISE | Master healer; protects against environmental pollutants; strengthens anatomy; guards against disease |
| | Communication; peace of mind; calming; loyalty; protective; restores healthy mental attitude |
| | Stone of friendship |
| ZIRCON | Self-esteem; strength; storing psychic power |

## *Selecting a Crystal or Gemstones*

Selecting the proper crystal is a very personal decision. The chart illustrates the common correspondences of crystals and gemstones, but part of making the right choice will depend on your personal energies.

You will need to open yourself to feel the powers or energies radiating from the crystal.

1.     Complete the grounding, centering, and shielding processes.

2.     Choose a crystal that you feel attracted to.

3.     Place the crystal in the palm of your right hand.

4.     Close your eyes and feel the crystal.

You might notice a variety of sensations from a change in temperature, a tingling, or an electrical current that illustrates that your energies and the crystal are attractants.

If you do not feel any change, select another crystal or gemstone appropriate for your task.

Continue until you locate a crystal or gemstone that causes you to feel a reaction.

5. When you have located a crystal that causes a reaction, think of the purpose you plan for the crystal and feel whether it is right for the job.

There is no way to describe how you will feel when you have selected the right crystal for a specific job. You will just know.

The most important factor is that you find a crystal that makes you feel an affinity.

Before you use the crystal you should cleanse it. The easiest way to cleanse a crystal is to expose it to direct sunlight.

I like to hold my crystal in the palm of my right hand and allow the rays of bright sunlight to cleanse it.

You could also cleanse your crystal in moonlight or by infusing it into the clean running water of a river or stream.

You should cleanse your crystal after each use.

# *Charging a Crystal or Gemstone*

A crystal consists of units of energy that align themselves in a specific manner. The crystal receives energy from the world around it, processes the energy and then transmits it back out into the world. This energy can be harnessed and directed by a skilled practitioner.

The crystal will gather energy on its own, but will be a more effective tool if you consistently charge it.

1.      Wash your crystal using soap and fresh, warm water.

2.      Rinse well with cool running water

3.      Place your crystal on a clear or reflective plate

4.      Place on the widow sill or another location where it can absorb early morning sun

5.      Carry the crystal with you throughout the day

6.      Return the crystal to the window sill where it can absorb early nighttime moonlight

7.      Carry the crystal with you throughout the night

8.      Return the crystal to the plate in the appropriate location any time you are not carrying it on your body

You will become familiar with the actions and emissions of your crystal so you will know both when it needs charged and when it is fully charged by how it feels to you.

## Energy Centers

Most natural therapies including spell work depend on the natural energies of the body and the elements for success. According to one philosophy, there are seven major psychic centers on the body called chakras enhanced by many minor chakras. The energy centers are also known as chi or ki.

Each of these energies centers form a link connecting the astral, mental, physical, and spiritual pathways of the body. These energies form a network of nerves and channels that follow the autonomic nervous system along the spinal cord.

These centers are believed to be magic power points where a person's energy is strongest. Energy can be channeled into these points to change person's emotional, mental, or physical levels.

The locations of each power point will vary by individual. The chakras give the most concise areas for beginning to locate each specific power point.

Crown Chakra    The crown chakra is located at the top of the head and corresponds with astral projection and enlightenment.

The energies of this chakra appear as violet white to many practitioners.

Heart Chakra    The heart chakra is located over the heart and corresponds with the element of air and with psychic touch.

The energies of this chakra appear as either green or bright pink to many practitioners.

Root Chakra    The root chakra is located at the base of the spine and relates to the element of earth and with psychic smell.

The energies of this chakra appear as a bright shade of red to many practitioners.

Sexual Chakra    The sexual chakra is located above the genitals and relates to the element of water and with psychic taste.

The energies of this chakra appear as a shade of orange to many practitioners.

Solar Plexus    The solar plexus chakra is located at the navel and corresponds with the element of fire and with psychic sight.

The energies of this chakra appear as a shade of bright yellow to many practitioners.

Third Eye    The third eye is located on the forehead between the eyes and is the center of psychic powers giving the ability to produce many psychic effects.

The energies of this chakra appear as a shade of deep blue to many practitioners.

Throat Chakra    The throat chakra is located at the base of the throat and corresponds with psychic hearing.

The energies of this chakra appear as a light shade of blue to many practitioners.

## *Locating Power Points*

Locating the power points on a person takes intuition on the part of the practitioner.

1.　You should ground and center yourself until you feel open and ready.

2.　Place your hands a few inches from the subject's body.

3.　Close your eyes and focus on how the energy from the person feels.

　　Remember this sensation because a change is indicative of a power point.

4.　Slowly begin to move your hands up and down the body keeping them a few inches from the surface.  Do not touch the person.

5.　You may feel a slight pulling or change in temperature between your hands and the body of the subject.

　　This is a power point.

　　　　The feeling of a power point will vary by practitioner and by subject.

　　　　You may feel a slight stickiness or electric charge or another sensation.

　　Any change from a lack of sensation indicates a likely power point for that person.

　　Allow yourself to be sensitive to any change from the baseline sensation you felt when you first placed your hands.

Helpful hints:  Stay relaxed.  You are trying to feel with your intuition, not think with your mind.  The more you allow your inner self to take charge of the process, the more success you will have in locating the energy points.

# *Auras*

Energy points give off certain specific colors but each individual has a certain color that surrounds them called an aura. An aura is an electromagnetic field that surrounds all living things. Some people are able to feel or sense an aura and others are actually able to see the aura of another person.

Auras are used to read a person's emotional and physical state. There is no specific way to read an aura that will work for everyone. Each individual has different characteristics that make certain processes easier for them than others.

1.      Begin by completing your grounding, centering, and shielding exercises

2.      Stand the person whose aura you are trying to read against a very dark or very light background. This is something that varies between individuals and you will want to try different approaches until you find the color that works best for you.

3.      Allow your eyes to go unfocused looking at the entire area around the person.

        This may take some practice. You need to counter your natural instinct to focus on a point.

4.      The aura in typically most clear around a person's head so attempt to keep the head within the field of vision near the person's head.

5.      The aura usually first becomes visible as a thin white film around the person.

6.       Continue to look beyond the white film. A secondary color should become visible.

# *General Aura Correspondences*

Blue            Idealistic, Imaginative, Intellectual, Spiritual

Crimson         Loyalty

Deep Red        Sensuality

Green           Compassion, Ingenuity, Growth

Maroon          Anger

Orange          Balance, Joy, Vitality

Pink            Cheer, Optimism

Purple          Spiritual Power

Red             Courage, Energy Strength

Yellow          Creativity, Spiritual, Wise

# CHAPTER 6

## Metal Correspondences

Metal is used to charge, to reflect, and as part of various spell craft. Like colors, gemstones, & crystals, metal has energies that make it more beneficial at some tasks than others.

You will find different metals correspond to certain practices you complete better than others do. This chart illustrates the most common metal correspondences. Your specific energies will dictate the correspondences that work best for you. As with any component, do not be afraid to vary from the norm and try working with various components.

ALUMINUM                        Powers Of Aluminum: A conductor of electricity.

BRASS                             Powers Of Brass: Healing; Money; Protection

Magic Uses: Brass can be used as a substitute for gold for money attracting
Magic rituals and spells.

Brass is used for sun Magic and fire Magic rituals and spells.

Because brass has protective attributes it is used for defensive Magic to protect and send back negativity to the sender.

COPPER

Powers Of Copper: Conductor of electricity; Healing; Love; Luck; Protection

Magic Uses: Copper is used to direct energy during ritual

Pure copper is worn for healing and to prevent sickness.

It is said that copper should be worn on the opposite side of your dominate hand.

Copper is also worn with emeralds to attract love

Copper is used to heal and prevent sickness because it has the ability to balance the polarities of the body

GOLD

Powers Of Gold: Power; Success; Wealth; Strength; Protection

Magic Uses: Used for sun spells and rituals to draw money and increase power, self-confidence or courage

Can be combined with white in protection spells

Worn on the body, gold helps to draw success and wealth

IRON

Powers of Iron: Protection; Healing; Strength

Magic Uses: Defensive magic to deflect negativity; psychic and emotional healing

A talisman of iron is said to increase strength when worn on the body

LEAD

Powers of Lead: Protection

Magic Uses: Used in defensive and protective magic to deflect negative energy.

Do not wear on the body

LODESTONE

Powers of Lodestone: Attraction – love, friendship, power, fidelity

Magic Uses: Lodestone is used for attraction magic

Lodestone is sometimes placed on the injured of the body in healing magic

Lodestone is usually carried in pairs

| SILVER | Power of Silver:  Intuition; Emotions; Psychic Mind; Dreams; Love; Protection |
|--------|--------|
| | Magic Uses;  Silver is used for water magic; divination; dreams; love; and healing spells |
| TIN | Power of Tin:  Money; Luck |
| | Magic Uses:  Used to create money drawing talismans |

## *Selecting Metal*

Selecting the proper metal for a specific need is a very personal decision.  The chart illustrates the common correspondences of different types of metal, but part of making the right choice will depend on your personal energies.

You will need to open yourself to feel the powers or energies radiating from the crystal.

1.      Complete the grounding, centering, and shielding processes.

2.      Choose a piece of metal that makes you feel an attraction.

3.      Place the metal in the palm of your right hand.

4.      Close your eyes and feel the metal.

You might notice a variety of sensations from a change in temperature, a tingling, or an electrical current that illustrates that your energies and the metal are attractants.

If you do not feel any change, select another piece or type of metal appropriate for your task.

Continue until you locate the metal that causes you to feel a reaction.

5.     When you have located the metal piece that causes a reaction, think of the purpose you plan for the metal and feel whether it is right for the job.

There is no way to describe how you will feel when you have selected the right metal for a specific job. You will just know.

The most important factor is that you find a piece of metal that makes you feel an affinity.

Before you use the metal for a specific purpose you should cleanse it. The easiest way to cleanse it is to expose it to direct sunlight. I like to hold my pieces of metal in the palm of my right hand and allow the rays of bright sunlight to cleanse it. You could also cleanse your metal pieces in moonlight or by infusing it into the clean running water of a river or stream. You should cleanse your metal after each use.

Metals consist of units of energy that align themselves in a specific manner. The metal receives energy from the world around it, processes the energy and then transmits it back out into the world. This energy can be harnessed and directed by a skilled practitioner.

The metal will gather energy on its own, but will be a more effective tool if you consistently charge it.

## How to Empower or Charge Metal

1.    Complete your grounding, centering, and shielding exercises

2.    Cleanse and empower your ingredients

3.    Wash your pieces of metal using soap and fresh, warm water.

4.    Rinse well with cool running water

5.    Place your metal on a clear or reflective plate

6.    Place on the widow sill or another location where it can absorb early morning sun

You will become familiar with the actions and emissions of your metal pieces so you will know both when it needs charged and when it is fully charged by how it feels to you.

**CHAPTER 7**

## Poppets and Dolls

Dolls and poppets have been used for positive and negative effect for generations. The healing doll is intended to bring peaceful tranquility to the recipient while stimulating the body's natural ability to heal itself.

Poppets are the most common and useful of the healing dolls, in fact, emotional and physical healing is the most common use for poppet dolls.

Poppets have many purposes and the intent of the maker is the most influential factor in the final effect of a poppet doll. You will also include various tools such as aromatic herbs, oils, talismans, and colors to help to direct the power of you doll.

Refer to the sections related to healing aromatics, color correspondences, metal correspondences, crystals, and gemstones to decide what items will be most effective at helping your poppet achieve your particular goals.

1.  Complete the grounding, centering, and shielding processes.

2.  Choose two fresh tree branches

3.  Thank the tree for its gifts

4.  Cross shape w/2 sticks

5.     Tie together w/hemp cord or waxed thread

6.     Wrap the stick with Spanish moss.

   ➢     Middle to head

   ➢     Down one arm

   ➢     Back across the other arm

   ➢     Back to the middle

   ➢     Down to the bottom

7.     Add herbs as you wind Spanish Moss

   You should use the herb appropriate for the goal you are trying to help effect

   Refer to the area related herbs blends and components that work well for your goal.

8.     Add parchment with the request you want the doll to fulfill written on it

9.     Wrap fabric strips around the moss – leave some showing at the head, ends of the arms, and the bottom of the legs

10.    Secure with a stitch or two of thread in a corresponding color

11.    Make a face – using beads, back eyed peas, or any other decorative items that you feel are suitable to the person and the needs

12. Dress the doll in one long strip of fabric whose color suits our ultimate goal.

    Refer to the section relating to color correspondences to help you select the color that will benefit you the most.

13. Wrap fabric around doll following the same path you used for the Spanish Moss

14. Add a string for hanging the doll where the recipient can see it and where it can be freshened by the sun and air

15. You should name the Poppet to represent the person who is to benefit from the healing spell

16. Should you be working for someone who has had surgery, then make an incision in the Poppet in the appropriate place.

17. Take the poppet from the altar and concentrate on the goal and direct your power into the patient as you sew up the incision.

## Distance Work

If you do not have access to the person who will be the recipient of the poppet, you will wish to complete an Auric healing using the Poppet in lieu of the actual person.

You need:

> A yellow candle

> Herbs blend that suits the desired goal.  If you do not know what herb blend will be most effective, you can refer to the section regarding Herb &

Oil Blends for ideas

- Clear quartz gemstone

- Photo or some part related to the person

- Perform on a Sunday.

- Stuff the doll with the herbs and add the gem about where the heart would be in the doll.

- Sew up the doll and do a naming ritual.

- Light the candle, and see the person healthy and happy in your mind.

- Say six times:

  Lavender, marigold, and rosemary

  The body, soul, and mind are free

  Stone of quartz, take the pain away

  Whole, healed, and free today

  With harm to none My will is done.

- Give the poppet to the person you are healing or if it was for yourself, keep it.

- If a binding was performed, then bury it off your property.

## Dream Pillows

Dream pillows have used in homeopathic and magical remedies for centuries. Each pillow is customized to the need of the recipient using colors, oils, and herbs designed to aid in healing a specific ailment, reenergizing the body to better equip it to win the battle against internal and external strife, or to aid the body and spirit in accomplishing a specific task.

You can make dream pillows in a variety of sizes and shapes to suit the decor of the room where they will be kept. I like to make mine the size of a standard throw pillow and mix varying pillows for varying needs. The pillow can be used as decor while providing a constant boost in energies. When used during rest, the pillow imbues the user with the healing powers that they need.

1.    Complete the grounding, centering, and shielding processes.

2.    Choose Two squares of fabric sized 12 ½ by 12 ½ for a standard throw pillow that you feel attracted to.

> You can use a differing size and shape if you have another end vision for your pillow.

> Some people like to use a symbolic print for their pillow. The print should mean something to the intended recipient.

> The best colors for healing are the colors the user associates with physical and mental health. If you are unsure of the colors you should

use select the one that best suits your goal from the listing in the section related to color correspondences.

2.   Place the fabric right sides facing each other.

3.   Sew three of the four sides

4.   You should have formed a sack.  Turn the sack inside right so that the pattern is facing outward.

5.   Add the herbs of your choice.  You can use the section related to Herb Blends to select your herbs or you could select the herbs from the chart below that best suits your goals.

6    Fill the pillow with a natural pre-made pillow form or hand fill with down

7.   You may wish to add a healing crystal, stone, or other symbol to the center of your pillow.

Refer to the section related to empowering and selecting your crystal for ideas on which one might work best for your particular need.

**CHAPTER**

**9**

# Charms, Talismans, and Amulets

Charms and amulets are used to channel certain energies toward or away from a person or particular area. They are usually combine attractants or repelling properties, which help to strengthen their goal. Just like metals, crystals, & gemstones, charms, talismans, & amulets will carry certain energies that you can channel toward your goal.

## *How to Select a Charm, Talisman, or Amulet*

Selecting the proper charm, talisman, or amulet components is a very personal decision. The most important factor in choosing the right charm, talisman, or amulet will be your personal energies.

You will need to open yourself to feel the powers or energies radiating from the items you intend to use in your ritual.

1.      Complete the grounding, centering, and shielding processes.

2.      Choose an item that you feel attracted to.

3.      Place the item in the palm of your right hand.

4.      Close your eyes and feel the item.

   ➢ You might notice a variety of sensations from a change in temperature, a tingling, or an electrical current that illustrates that your energies and the item are attractants.

> If you do not feel any change, select another item appropriate for your task.

> Continue until you locate an item that causes you to feel a reaction.

5.  When you have located an appropriate item that causes a reaction, think of the purpose you plan for the item and feel whether it is right for the job.

There is no way to describe how you will feel when you have selected the right items for a specific job.  You will just know.

The most important factor is that you find an item that makes you feel an affinity.

## How to Empower a Charm, Talisman, or Amulet

1.  Complete your grounding, centering, and shielding exercises

2.  Cleanse and empower your ingredients

3.  Wash your item if necessary and possible using soap and fresh, warm water.

4.  Rinse well with cool running water

5.  Place your item on a clear or reflective plate

6   Place on the widow sill or another location where it can absorb early morning sun

You will become familiar with the actions and emissions of your charms, amulets, & talismans so you will know both when they need charged and when they are fully charged by how they feel to you.

**CHAPTER 10**

# Aromatics

There are many ways to use herbs & oils in spell craft. Some of the most effective are those that keep the herb & oil blend on or near the person. We use aromatic bags, dream pillows, mojo bags, anointing oils, and spritzs as ways to infuse the air with the beneficial elements of each blend.

## *Aromatic Jars*

1. Complete your grounding, centering, and shielding exercises

2. Cleanse and empower your ingredients

3. Gather:    ¼ cup +/-    Baking Soda

                   4 tsp +/-    Herb Blend of Choice

4. Fill the jar ¾ of the way full with baking soda

5. Top with crushed herbs of your choice.

6. Place jars on shelves around the house

If the scent seems to be fading, stir the herbs gently with the tip of your finger to release the smell.

# Aromatic Bags

1. Complete your grounding, centering, and shielding exercises

2. Cleanse and empower your ingredients

3. Create a       Drawstring Bag     1 ½ inch x 1 ½ inch

   ➢ You can make this bag by cutting a rectangle 3 x 1 ½ inches

   ➢ Fold the rectangle in ½ with the printed side facing inward

   ➢ Stitch the sides of the bag

   ➢ Fold ¼ inch down at the top of the bag

   ➢ Sew all but the last ½ inch of the bag

   ➢ Run a cord through the pocket you created with the seam

   ➢ Turn the bag inside out

4. Fill the bag with the aromatic herb of your choice

5. Pull the drawstring to close the bag

6. Place the bag in your pocket, under your pillow, or in another accessible place

7. Periodically, open the bag and inhale the aromatic blend

# *Aromatic Blend Spray*

1.  Complete your grounding, centering, and shielding exercises

2.  Cleanse and empower your ingredients

3.  Gather        1 cup        Water

    Aromatic Blend of Choice

4.  Blend herbs and water in a medium sauce pan.

5.  Bring the mixture to a light boil.

6.  Reduce heat and simmer for approximately 30-45 minutes

7.  Allow to cool.

8.  Add        1 cup        Witch Hazel

9.  Pour into your preferred spray bottle.

10. Shake well

11. Spray on your hair and skin, in the air, on soft furnishings and fabrics, on carpet and floors, and any place else where the scents will surround you.

# *Aromatic Simmer*

1.  Complete your grounding, centering, and shielding exercises

2.  Cleanse and empower your ingredients

3.  Gather     2 cups     Water

    ¼ cup     White Vinegar

    ¼ cup     Herb Blend of Choice

4.  Place all of the ingredients in a small saucepan or simmer pot

5.  Simmer on low heat

6.  Add more water as needed

## Spells to Draw Good Luck

Luck is one example of a characteristic that some people are believed to have in abundance and that others attempt to attain through spell casting. We have all heard someone say "They are so lucky" about another person.

Luck, like anything, is dependent on many factors. You can help to channel the natural world to increase your luck, but you must also believe in yourself and your ability to BE lucky.

Belief in self is the first, and most important, ingredient in good luck work. In fact, belief in your ability to channel the natural world to achieve your goals is the most important ingredient to success in any endeavor.

The suggested rituals, blends, and instructions on the following pages are just that suggestions based on the most effective steps we take to meet the needs of those who come to us seeking aide. As long as your intent is true and your belief in yourself is strong, these should work well for you. If you find yourself having difficulty with any instruction included, take time to ground, center yourself, and then meditate for a time on what you might do to adapt the inclusions so that they are better suited to your personal energies & abilities. The correspondences charts throughout this book might assist you in adapting the spell craft to meet your needs.

## Good Luck Plants

Calamus Brings luck to the gardener

## Lucky Oil Bottle

1.  Complete your grounding, centering, and shielding exercises

2.  Fill a tall, thin bottle ½ way with

    | | |
    |---|---|
    | 3 drops | clove oil |
    | 3 drops | violet oil |
    | 3 drops | yellow colorant |

3.  Cleanse and empower your ingredients

4.  Mix

    | | |
    |---|---|
    | 3 tbsp | water |
    | 1/3 tsp | cinnamon |
    | 1/3 tsp | nutmeg |
    | 3 drops | red colorant |

5.  Fill jar to the top with red mixture

6.  The red mixture will separate from the yellow mixture

7.  Each day, shake the mixture well and sprinkle a few drops around the house or in your hair

## Lucky Feet Balm

This balm should be applied to your feet each day before you leave the house. It will attract good luck to you.

1.    Complete your grounding, centering, and shielding exercises

2.    Gather        1 tbsp        lotion base of choice

                    1 tsp         olive oil

                    3 drops       jasmine oil

                    1 tsp         nutmeg

                    1 tsp         parsley

3.    Cleanse and empower your ingredients

4.    Blend ingredients well

5.    Anoint feet before leaving the house


## Nutmeg Luck Attractant Amulet

1.    Complete your grounding, centering, and shielding exercises

2.    Cleanse and empower your ingredients

3.    Drill a hole in the nut

4.    Fill the hole with liquid tin

5.    Seal the hole with wax

6.    Carry with you at all times

## Lucky Hand Balm

Anoint your hands with this balm many times throughout the day and especially when you will be gambling or meeting those who can bring you good fortune.

1. Complete your grounding, centering, and shielding exercises

2. Gather
   | | | |
   |---|---|---|
   | 3 tbsp | lotion base of choice |
   | 1 tsp | olive oil |
   | 1 tsp | cinnamon |
   | 1 tsp | dried chamomile |
   | 1 tsp | nutmeg |

3. Cleanse and empower your ingredients

4. Blend ingredients well

5. Anoint hands daily, whenever you are gambling, or whenever you are meeting a person who might bring good fortune into your life

# Good Luck Herb Jar

This jar will attract good luck and help to change bad luck to good

1.      Complete your grounding, centering, and shielding exercises

2.      Gather     1 tsp   chamomile

                   1 tsp   clover

                   1 tsp   frankincense

                   1 tsp   Irish moss

                   1 tsp   mistletoe

                   1 tsp   holly

3.      Cleanse and empower your ingredients

4.      Stir the herbs well

5.      Seal the jar and place it on a windowsill in where it will receive bright sunlight & moonlight

6.      Shake the jar each morning and then open to inhale the aroma

7.      Seal the jar and put it back on the widow sill

8.      Replace your herbs each month or whenever the beneficial effects seem to be fading from your life

## Good Luck Attractant Charm

Every facet of this charm is designed to help attract good luck to the person who carries it with respect.

1. Complete your grounding, centering, and shielding exercises

2. Gather
   | | |
   |---|---|
   | 1 | yellow flannel bag |
   | 3 | all spice berries |
   | 1 tsp | bistort |
   | 1 tsp | galangal |
   | 1 tsp | nutmeg |

3. Cleanse and empower your ingredients

4. Place all of the ingredients in the bag

5. Shake the bag each morning

6. Inhale the scents

7. Carry with you to attract luck

## Gamblers Luck Charm

1.      Complete your grounding, centering, and shielding exercises

2.      Gather     1              red flannel bag
                   1 tsp          ginger
                   1 tsp          lucky hand
                   1 tsp          nutmeg

3.      Cleanse and empower your ingredients

4.      Place all of the ingredients in the bag

5.      Shake the bag each morning

6.      Inhale the scents

7.      Carry with you to attract luck


## Lucky Amulet Bag

1.      Complete your grounding, centering, and shielding exercises

2.      Gather     1              small bag of choice
                   3              pieces fresh straw
                   3              job's tears seeds
                   3              mustard seeds
                   3              holly leaves
                   3              olive leaves

3.      Cleanse and empower your ingredients

4.      Place all of the items in your bag

5.      Carry with you at all times to attract good luck

## House Amulet for Good Luck

1.  Complete your grounding, centering, and shielding exercises

2.  Gather     3         aloe leaves

              3         holly branches

              18        pieces of straw

              1         bamboo stalk

3.  Cleanse and empower your ingredients

4.  Twine the aloe, holly, and straw around the bamboo.
5.  Hang above the doorway in your home to attract good luck and keeps the energy flowing

## Lucky Cabinet Amulet

1.  Complete your grounding, centering, and shielding exercises

2.  Gather     1         yellow bag

              3 tbsp     alfalfa

3.  Cleanse and empower your ingredients

4.  Keep the bag in your cabinet to draw good luck to the home

# Home Sachet Bag for Luck

This amulet bag can be kept in the home to draw good luck and protect from negativity

1. Complete your grounding, centering, and shielding exercises

2. Gather 1 yellow flannel bag

   1 tsp wood rose

   1 tsp thyme

   1 tsp ground orange rind

   1 tsp myrtle

   1 tsp bayberry

3. Cleanse and empower your ingredients

4. Place the herbs inside the flannel bag

5. Hang in the home

6. Shake the bag each morning and night to attract luck

## *Fast Luck Charm*

1.    Complete your grounding, centering, and shielding exercises

2.    Gather:      1              aventurine

         1/3 tsp        nutmeg

         1/3 tsp        allspice

         1/3 tsp        cinnamon

3.    Cleanse and empower your ingredients

4.    Hold the aventurine in one hand

5.    See what changes in your luck could do to your life.

6.    Sprinkle the cinnamon, nutmeg, and allspice on the aventurine.

7.    Say

      Aventurine, bring me good luck.
      May my luck change from this day forward
      Aventurine bring me good luck

8.    Keep your charm on you at all times.

9.    If your luck doesn't change after a few weeks, recharge the charm again with this spell.

## Lucky Candle Blend

As you become more adept at formulating your own spell craft and gain a deeper understanding of the properties of different herbs and oils you will want to formulate custom blends that work well for you.  This recipe is one of the most effective blends for the most common requests we receive from people seeking aide.

| 1 cup | melted candle base |
| 9 drops | green colorant |
| 6 drops | cedar oil |
| 6 drops | almond oil |
| 6 drops | basil oil |
| 6 drops | clove oil |
| 6 drops | coconut oil |

# Lucky Herb & Oil Blends

These are some of the most effective herb & oil blends we use for the most common requests from people who seek aide. You can use these herbs & oils in poppets, dream pillows, candles, mojo bags, simmers, sprays, and sachets. You can also incorporate the blends into spells of your own design for additional powers.

There are many decent guides on herb and oil blends similar to my **Compendium of Beneficial Herbs & Oils.** As you advance in the craft, you will wish to obtain a guide of expanded herbs & oils, their properties, side effects, and use from a reputable source. The expanded guides will help you in creating your own spell craft and remedies.

## Fast Luck Blend

| | |
|---|---|
| 1 tbsp | alfalfa |
| 1 tbsp | all spice berries |
| 1 tbsp | cedar chips |
| 1 tbsp | ginger |

## Luck Attracting Oil

| | |
|---|---|
| 3 drops | clove oil |
| 3 drops | violet oil |
| 1 tbsp | carrier oil such as jojoba or coconut |

Blend well

Store in an airtight container

## Good Luck Blend

½ cup        chamomile tea

½ cup        pineapple juice

½ cup        queen of the meadow tea

Add to the bath and soak at least 30 minutes to draw good luck.  Do not rinse.


## Good Luck, Fortune, & Prosperity House Wash

Added to your floor wash, this helps to draw good luck, good fortune, & prosperity to the home

1 tsp        wisteria oil

1 tsp        patchouli oil

1 tsp        juniper oil

1 tsp        cinnamon

1 gallon     hot water


## Good Luck Home or Business Spray

8 drops      basil oil

8 drops      cedar oil

8 drops      peppermint oil

## Gambler's Blend

1 tsp        chamomile

1 tsp        cinnamon

1 tsp        ginger

## Potpourri to Draw Good Luck & Protect from Negative Energies

3 tbsp      juniper berries

3 tbsp      basil

3 tbsp      frankincense

3 tbsp      crushed dill seeds

3 tbsp      crushed clove

3 tbsp      shredded bay leaves

Blend herbs well and place in small bowls or jars around them home to draw good luck and protect from negative energies

# CHAPTER 12

## Prosperity and Money Spells

Money is an example something that we all need to survive. One of the most important rules of prosperity and money spells is that you should always balance your requests with your needs. In order to make money & prosperity spells work well for you, you must respect the nature of magic. Keep the request reasonable and keep your intent pure and your requests will be answered.

The suggested rituals, blends, and instructions on the following pages are just that suggestions based on the most effective steps we take to meet the needs of those who come to us seeking aide. As long as your intent is true and your belief in yourself is strong, these should work well for you. If you find yourself having difficulty with any instruction included, take time to ground, center yourself, and then meditate for a time on what you might do to adapt the inclusions so that they are better suited to your personal energies & abilities. The correspondences charts throughout this book might assist you in adapting the spell craft to meet your needs.

## Money Knot Spell

1. Complete your grounding, centering, and shielding exercises

2. Gather      3 lengths of a silk, cord, or ribbon

         1      deep green

         1      yellow or gold

         1      light green

     approximately each 9-12 inches in length

3. Cleanse and empower your ingredients

4. Braid the lengths of cord together until you have one long piece

5. Tie 9 knots in the braid while saying

     Tie knot 1 while saying

         By knot of one, my spell's begun

     Tie knot 2 while saying

         By knot of two, plenty fruitful work to do

     Tie knot 3 while saying

         By knot of three, money comes to me

     Tie knot 4 while saying

         By knot of four, opportunity knocks at my door

     Tie knot 5 while saying

         By knot of five, my business thrives

Tie knot 6 while saying

> By knot of six, this spell is fixed

Tie knot 7 while saying

> By knot of seven, success is given

Tie knot 8 while saying

> By knot of eight, increase is great

Tie knot 9 while saying

> By knot of nine, these things are mine

6.  Use the cord as a bracelet, carry the cord with you, or wear it as a necklace amulet cord


## *Prosperity Mojo Bag*

1.  Complete your grounding, centering, and shielding exercises

2.  Gather    1        leather drawstring bag

              3 tbsp    chopped alfalfa

              3 tbsp    chopped bayberry

              3 tbsp    chamomile
3.  Cleanse and empower your ingredients

4.  Mix herbs & place inside bag

5.  Carry with you

6.  Shake herbs & inhale scent daily

### Money Anointing Spell

1.     Complete your grounding, centering, and shielding exercises

2.     Gather     1 drop     cedar oil

                  1 drop     pine oil

                  1 drop     almond oil

                  1 drop     bergamot oil

                  Money

3.     Cleanse and empower your ingredients

4.     Anoint the money in your wallet with 1 drop of each oil daily to attract more money


### Prosperity Mojo Bag

1.     Complete your grounding, centering, and shielding exercises

2.     Gather     1           leather drawstring bag

                  3 tbsp     chopped alfalfa

                  3 tbsp     chopped bayberry

                  3 tbsp     chamomile

3.     Cleanse and empower your ingredients

4.     Mix herbs & place inside bag

5.     Carry with you

6.     Shake herbs & inhale scent daily

## Prosperity Conjure Bag

This conjure bag aids you in finding money

1.  Complete your grounding, centering, and shielding exercises

2.  Gather      1              small green bag or packet

              1              lodestone (magnet)

              1 tsp      smartweed

              1 tsp      cinnamon

              1 tbsp    gold sand

3.  Cleanse and empower your ingredients

4.  Place the magnet and smartweed in the bag

5.  Feed your bag a pinch of gold sand every day until you have found the money that you need

## Dollar Amulet

1.      Complete your grounding, centering, and shielding exercises

2.      Gather      1      dollar bill

                    1      length of green wire, cord, or ribbon

                    1      almond

                    1      sprig alfalfa

3.      Cleanse and empower your ingredients

4,      Roll the herbs inside the money

5.      Tie the roll closed with the wire, cord, or ribbon

6.      Put the bill somewhere it will not be bothered inside your purse or home

## Money Powder

1.      Complete your grounding, centering, and shielding exercises

2.      Gather      1 tbsp      powdered cedar

                    1 tbsp      powdered sweet basil

                    1 tbsp      powdered dill seeds

                    1 tbsp      cinnamon

3.      Cleanse and empower your ingredients

4.      Blend all of the powders well

5.      Rub your money with this powder before you spend it to draw your money back to you and to help it attract other people's money on the way!

## Fast Prosperity Charm

1.   Complete your grounding, centering, and shielding exercises

2.   Gather:   1          tiger's eye

              1/3 tsp    thistle

              1/3 tsp    sweet pea

              1/3 tsp    strawberry

3.   Cleanse and empower your ingredients

4.   Cast the circle. Hold the tiger's eye in one hand

5.   Meditate for a few moments, see yourself, and see what your financial blessings could do in your life.

6.   Sprinkle the basil, sage and the orange oil on the tiger's eye.

7.   Say these words

     Tiger's Eye, bring me good prosperity.

     May my luck change from this day forward

     Tiger's Eye bring me financial blessings

8.   Close the circle

9.   Keep the charm with you at all times

## Money Poppet or Doll Blend

1.  Complete your grounding, centering, and shielding exercises

2.  Cleanse and empower your ingredients

3.  Create a poppet using green

4.  Sew a small piece of gold or tin inside the doll

5.  Add the beneficial herb or oil blend that suits your needs

6.  Obtain two green candles

7.  Anoint the candles with the appropriate oil blend for your needs

8.  Set the doll between the candles

9.  Light the candles

10. Meditate and think of the money that you need

## Money Attractant Bag

Use this bag to increase luck and ensure a steady flow of money

1.  Complete your grounding, centering, and shielding exercises

2.  Gather    1          green flannel bag

             1 tbsp     peony

             1 tbsp     chopped moss

             3          acorns

3.  Cleanse and empower your ingredients

4.  Place all of the items in the bag and carry it with you to increase your luck and ensure a steady flow of money. Sleep with the bag under your pillow at night.


## Wallet Prosperity Charm

1.  Complete your grounding, centering, and shielding exercises

2.  Gather    1          small yellow bag or packet

             3          cedar chips

             3          flax seeds

             3          slices ginger

3.  Cleanse and empower your ingredients

4.  Place in a small yellow bag or packet

5.  Carry in your purse or wallet to attract money

## House Money Attracting Bag

1.  Complete your grounding, centering, and shielding exercises

2.  Gather

    | | | |
    |---|---|---|
    | 1 | | leather bag |
    | 3 tbsp | | alfalfa |
    | 3 tbsp | | moss |
    | 3 tbsp | | nutmeg |
    | 1 | | mandrake root – whole |
    | 1 | | galangal root |
    | 3 pieces | | silver |

3.  Cleanse and empower your ingredients

4.  Place all of the items in the bag

5.  Keep the bag in the most used room of your home to increase luck, attract prosperity, and ensure a steady flow of money into the home

## Wallet or Purse Oils

1. Complete your grounding, centering, and shielding exercises

2. Gather     1         small jar

                  3 drops    heather oil

                  3 drops    mint oil

                  1 tsp      almond oil

3. Cleanse and empower your ingredients

4. Blend oils well

5. Pour into jar and seal tightly

6. Rub a few drops of oil into your wallet or purse daily to draw money


## House Money Amulet

1. Complete your grounding, centering, and shielding exercises

2. Gather     1         small green packet

                  1         sprig of sarsaparilla

                  1         sprig of thyme

                  1         magnet

                  3         small coins

3. Cleanse and empower your ingredients

4. Place the amulet above the doorway you use to enter your home to invite in prosperity.

## Prosperity Amulet

1.  Complete your grounding, centering, and shielding exercises

2.  Gather:    One thin gold band
    One thin copper band
    One thin silver band

3.  Cleanse and empower your ingredients

4.  On the index finger of your left hand

    place the gold band

    place the copper band

    place the silver band.

5.  When you wish to have good fortune turn the bands clockwise and focus all of you energies on drawing the energies of fortune toward you


## Money Hands

1.  Complete your grounding, centering, and shielding exercises

2.  Gather    1 tbsp    lotion base of choice
    1 tsp    powdered bergamot
    1 tsp    powdered dill seeds
    1 tsp    powdered thyme
    3 drops    cedar oil

3.  Cleanse and empower your ingredients

4.  Blend ingredients well

5.  Anoint hands before leaving the house

## Wallet Charm

1.   Complete your grounding, centering, and shielding exercises

2.   Gather     1          small green packet or bag

                    1          unshelled almond or acorn

                    3          dill seeds

                    1 tsp      cinnamon

                    1 tsp      honeysuckle

3.   Cleanse and empower your ingredients

4.   Place all of the items inside the green bag or packet.

5.   Carry the packet in your wallet or purse to attract money

## Money Box

1.   Complete your grounding, centering, and shielding exercises

2.   Gather     1          small box
                    3 tbsp    herb blend of choice
                    3 pieces   lodestone

3.   Cleanse and empower your ingredients

4.   Place the ingredients inside the box

5.   Close the box and seal the top

     Do not seal all of the edges since you want the herbs to attract money

6.   Whenever you are in need of money, shake the box while concentrating on your need

## *Money Bottle*

1.    Complete your grounding, centering, and shielding exercises

2.    Fill a tall, thin bottle ½ way with

      3 drops      cedar oil

      3 drops      pine oil

      3 drops      patchouli oil

3.    Cleanse and empower your ingredients

4.    Fill the remaining space in the jar with

          almond Oil

      3 drops      red colorant

5.    The red mixture will separate from the yellow mixture

6.    Each day, shake the mixture well and sprinkle a few drops around the house or in your hair

# *Money Jar*

1. Complete your grounding, centering, and shielding exercises

2. Gather    pen

           3 x 3 piece of paper

           jar with tight fitting lid

           7 pieces of gold or tin

           herb blend suitable to your needs

3. Cleanse and empower your ingredients

4. Write your need on the paper and drop it into the jar

5. Drop the 7 pieces of gold or tin into the jar using your right hand

6. As each piece of metal drops, visualize it multiplying

7. As each piece drops say

   With this wish, my money grows
   night and day it overflows
   in moonlight or sunshine
   come to me now, you are mine

8. Inhale the fragrance of the herbs you have selected

9. Sprinkle the herbs over the wish and money

10. Seal the jar tightly and place it where you can see it every day

11. Feed a coin or two and more of your herb blend to the jar each morning and night

12. After you obtain the money that you need, remove the paper from the jar and bury it near your back door

# Prosperity & Money Candle Blends

As you become more adept at formulating your own spell craft and gain a deeper understanding of the properties of different herbs and oils you will want to formulate custom blends that work well for you. These recipes are some of the most effective blends for the most common requests we receive from people seeking aide.

## Money Attractant Candle

| 1 cup | melted candle base |
|-------|--------------------|
| 9 drops | green colorant |
| 1 ½ tsp | all spice |
| 1½ tsp | almond |
| 1½ tsp | basil |
| 1 ½ tsp | bergamot |
| 1 ½ tsp | cloves |

## Prosperity & Wealth Candle

| 1 cup | melted candle base |
|-------|--------------------|
| 9 drops | green colorant |
| 6 drops | almond oil |
| 6 drops | bayberry oil |
| 1 ½ tsp | basil |
| 1 ½ tsp | pine needles |

# Prosperity & Money Herb & Oil Blends

These are some of the most effective herb & oil blends we use for the most common requests from people who seek aide. You can use these herbs & oils in poppets, dream pillows, candles, mojo bags, simmers, sprays, and sachets. You can also incorporate the blends into spells of your own design for additional powers.

There are many decent guides on herb and oil blends similar to my **Compendium of Beneficial Herbs & Oils.** As you advance in the craft, you will wish to obtain a guide of expanded herbs & oils, their properties, side effects, and use from a reputable source. The expanded guides will help you in creating your own spell craft and remedies.

## Fast Money Blend

| | |
|---|---|
| ½ tsp | all spice |
| ½ tsp | almond |
| ½ tsp | basil |
| ½ tsp | bergamot |
| ½ tsp | cloves |

## Money Attractant Blend

| | |
|---|---|
| 1 tbsp | comfrey |
| 1 tbsp | chamomile |
| 1 tbsp | nutmeg |
| 3 tbsp | crushed dill seeds |

## Prosperity Blend

6 drops     cedar oil

6 drops     almond oil

6 drops     basil oil

6 drops     clove oil

6 drops     coconut oil

## Good Luck, Fortune & Prosperity House Wash

Added to your floor wash, this helps to draw good luck, good fortune, & prosperity to the home

1 tsp     wisteria oil

1 tsp     patchouli oil

1 tsp     juniper oil

1 tsp     cinnamon

1 gallon     hot water

## Money Oil

10 drops     almond

10 drops     bergamot

## Money Attractant Powder or Incense

| | |
|---|---|
| 3 tsp | powdered almond |
| 3 tsp | powdered all spice |
| 3 tsp | powdered basil |
| 3 tsp | powdered clove |
| 3 tsp | orange oil |

Mix powders well

Blend in orange oils

Add to incense or blend powders into ½ cup baking soda to use as a carpet sprinkle

## Prosperity, Happiness & Protection Blend

| | |
|---|---|
| 1 tbsp | allspice |
| 1 tbsp | almond |
| 1 tbsp | cinnamon |
| 3 drops | lime juice |

## Job & Confidence Spells

Confidence is one example of a characteristic that some people are believed to have in abundance and that others attempt to attain through spell casting.

Self-Confidence, like anything, is dependent on many factors. You can help to channel the natural world to increase your sense of confidence especially when it comes to attracting a job, but you must also believe in yourself.

Belief in self is the first, and most important, ingredient in spell work. In fact, belief in your ability to channel the natural world to achieve your goals is the most important ingredient to success in any endeavor.

The suggested rituals, blends, and instructions on the following pages are just that suggestions based on the most effective steps we take to meet the needs of those who come to us seeking aide. As long as your intent is true and your belief in yourself is strong, these should work well for you. If you find yourself having difficulty with any instruction included, take time to ground, center yourself, and then meditate for a time on what you might do to adapt the inclusions so that they are better suited to your personal energies & abilities. The correspondences charts throughout this book might assist you in adapting the spell craft to meet your needs.

## *Job Oil Bottle*

1.  Complete your grounding, centering, and shielding exercises

2.  Fill a tall, thin bottle ½ way with

    3 drops      bergamot oil

    3 drops      jasmine oil

    3 drops      yellow colorant

3.  Cleanse and empower your ingredients

4.  Mix

    3 tbsp       water

    1/3 tsp      lemon balm

    1/3 tsp      rosemary

    3 drops      purple colorant

5.  Fill jar to the top with purple mixture

6.  The purple mixture will separate from the yellow mixture

7.  Each day, shake the mixture well and sprinkle a few drops in your hair or on your briefcase that you will carry to the interview

## Job Seekers Knot Spell

1.    Complete your grounding, centering, and shielding exercises

2.    Gather    3 lengths of a silk, cord, or ribbon
            1      deep green
            1      yellow or gold
            1      red

      approximately each 9-12 inches in length

3.    Cleanse and empower your ingredients

4.    Braid the lengths of cord together until you have one long piece

5.    Tie 9 knots in the braid while saying

      Tie knot 1 while saying

            By knot of one, my spell's begun

      Tie knot 2 while saying

            By knot of two, plenty fruitful work to do

      Tie knot 3 while saying

            By knot of three, money comes to me

      Tie knot 4 while saying

            By knot of four, opportunity knocks at my door

      Tie knot 5 while saying

            By knot of five, my business thrives

      Tie knot 6 while saying

By knot of six, this spell is fixed

Tie knot 7 while saying

By knot of seven, success is given

Tie knot 8 while saying

By knot of eight, increase is great

Tie knot 9 while saying

By knot of nine, these things are mine


6.      Use the cord as a bracelet, carry the cord with you, or wear it as a
        necklace amulet cord


## *Job Seekers Hand Balm*

1.      Complete your grounding, centering, and shielding exercises

2.      Gather        1 tbsp         lotion base of choice

                       1 tsp          olive oil

                       3 drops        jasmine oil

                       3 drops        musk

                       3 drops        ylang-ylang

3.      Cleanse and empower your ingredients

4.      Blend ingredients well

5.      Anoint hands before leaving the house

## Interview Luck Bag

This jar will attract good luck or change bad luck to good

1.      Complete your grounding, centering, and shielding exercises

2.      Gather       1 tbsp        crushed almonds

                     3 drops       rose oil

                     3 drops       jasmine oil

                     3 drops       ylang-ylang

                     1 jar         with tight lid

                     1             small purple bag

3.      Cleanse and empower your ingredients

4.      Place the crushed nuts in the jar

5.      Pour the oils over the nuts

5.      Seal the jar and place it on a windowsill in where it will receive bright sunlight & moonlight

6.      Shake the jar each morning and then open to inhale the aroma

7.      Seal the jar and put it back on the widow sill

8.      After three nights, pour the mixture into the bag

9.      Carry the bag with you to interviews

## Confidence Spell

1. Find a stone that resembles a lion's head. You can buy a charm if you prefer.

2. Light a yellow candle

3. Pass the charm through the flame of the candle three times

4. While you pass the charm through the candle flame, think about your good points and the respect you deserve

5. Anoint the candle with the oil blend that makes you feel calm and confident. If you do not have a preferred blend, you can use the appropriate blend from the section on herb & oil blends

6. Put the charm on a chain or cord and wear it on a chain or put it in your pocket.

7. Whenever you touch it, feel the confidence building within you.

## Job Attractant Charm

1. Complete your grounding, centering, and shielding exercises

2. Gather    1    red flannel bag
           3    all spice berries
           1 tsp   kava kava
           1 tsp   lemon balm

3. Cleanse and empower your ingredients

4. Place all of the ingredients in the bag

5. Shake the bag each morning & Inhale the scents

7. Carry with you to interviews to attract the job you want

## *Job Charm*

1.  Complete your grounding, centering, and shielding exercises

2.  Gather:     1            alexandrite

               3 drops      rosemary oil

               3 drops      musk

               3 drops      lemon balm

3.  Cleanse and empower your ingredients

4.  Hold the alexandrite in one hand

5.  See what changes this job will bring to your life.

6.  Sprinkle the oils on the alexandrite.

7.  Say

    Alexandrite, bring me this job.
    May my life change from this day forward
    alexandrite bring me this job

8.  Keep your charm on you at all times.

9.  If you do not get the job you need, recharge the charm again with this spell.

# Self Improvement Spell

1.  Gather

    ➢ Wooden Clothespin

    ➢ Black Felt Marker

    ➢ Small Pieces of Paper

    ➢ Pin

    ➢ Black Pepper

2.  Cleanse and empower your ingredients

3.  Use the marker to write the bad habits you want to break on the slips of paper

4.  Place each slip of paper inside the clothespin

5.  Sit quietly and meditate on changes you wish to occur.

6.  When you are finished thinking about the changes say

    "This spell I do, within my rights to be free~
    Darken my house no more! Begone! Begone from me!"

7.  Sprinkle the clothespin and papers with

8.  Bury the clothespin near your front door.

## Interview Confidence & Job Seeking Success

## Herb & Oil Blends

These are some of the most effective herb & oil blends we use for the most common requests from people who seek aide. You can use these herbs & oils in poppets, dream pillows, candles, mojo bags, simmers, sprays, and sachets. You can also incorporate the blends into spells of your own design for additional powers.

There are many decent guides on herb and oil blends similar to my **Compendium of Beneficial Herbs & Oils.** As you advance in the craft, you will wish to obtain a guide of expanded herbs & oils, their properties, side effects, and use from a reputable source. The expanded guides will help you in creating your own spell craft and remedies.

### Interview Luck Blend

| | |
|---|---|
| 1 tbsp | apple blossom |
| 1 tbsp | bergamot |
| 1 tbsp | lemon balm |

### Job Attracting Oil

| | |
|---|---|
| 3 drops | ylang-ylang |
| 3 drops | musk |
| 1 tbsp | carrier oil such as jojoba or coconut |

Blend well

Store in an airtight container

## Job Seekers Blend – to help you gain the job you want

| | |
|---|---|
| 8 drops | all spice oil |
| 8 drops | rosemary oil |
| 8 drops | sage |
| 8 drops | ginger oil |

## Confidence Inspiring Blend to give you strength and courage

| | |
|---|---|
| 8 drops | bergamot oil |
| 8 drops | rosemary oil |
| 8 drops | lavender |

## Potpourri to Draw Good Luck & Protect from Negative Energies

| | |
|---|---|
| 3 tbsp | juniper berries |
| 3 tbsp | basil |
| 3 tbsp | frankincense |
| 3 tbsp | crushed dill seeds |
| 3 tbsp | crushed clove |
| 3 tbsp | shredded bay leaves |

Blend herbs well and place in small bowls or jars around them home to draw good luck and protect from negative energies

## Job Luck Bath Bag

Use daily to change your luck, enhance personal protection from negativity, injury, and harm and to increase the likelihood of getting the job you want

| | |
|---|---|
| 1 tsp | basil |
| 1 tsp | bay |
| 1 tsp | chamomile |
| 1 tsp | rosemary |

## Daytime Confidence Inspiring Scented Candle

| | |
|---|---|
| 6 drops | all spice oil |
| 6 drops | rosemary oil |
| 6 drops | sage |
| 6 drops | ginger oil |
| 9 drops | colorant – red |
| 1 cup | candle wax base |

**CHAPTER**

**14**

## Business Spells

Many people want to own their own business or make more sales at their current job. Just as each person is different, each business and job is different. This is a section where you might want to let your creativity and the knowledge you have gained run free. These spells are designed to generally help you draw more customers to your business and to encourage each customer to spend more money. The herb correspondences section at the end has many, many herbs & oils that may be beneficial to your business needs in a way they are not to another. You should customize the inclusions in each instructional to suit your specific business goals & needs.

### *Thriving Business Plant*

A thriving Sage plant will cause the business to thrive as long as it lives

## Business Bells

1.  Complete your grounding, centering, and shielding exercises

2.  Gather     1      yellow flannel bag
                  3      sprigs of mistletoe
                  1 tsp   dried mint
                  1 tsp   dried peony flowers

3.  Cleanse and empower your ingredients

4.  Place all of the ingredients in the bag

5.  Hang the bag above the door to attract customers and success to the business

## Door Knob Wash

1.  Complete your grounding, centering, and shielding exercises

2.  Gather     7 drops      yellow dock root

                    7 drops      citronella oil

                    7 drops      clover oil

                    3 tbsp      almond oil

3.  Cleanse and empower your ingredients

4.  Blend the oils well

5.  Pour into a jar with a tightly fitting lid

6.  Wipe the doorknobs of your business with the oils each morning to attract customers to your door

## *Business Amulet*

1.    Complete your grounding, centering, and shielding exercises

2.    Gather:      1          garnet

              3 drops    citronella oil

              3 drops    mint oil

              3 drops    clover oil

3.    Cleanse and empower your ingredients

4.    Hold the garnet in one hand

5.    See what changes a thriving business could bring to your life.

6.    Sprinkle the oils on the garnet.

7.    Say

Garnet, please, bring me success.

May my life change from this day forward

Garnet, please, bring me success

8.    Keep your charm on you or at the place of business at all times.

9.    If your does not improve as much as you need, recharge the charm again with this spell.

## Thriving Business Mojo Bag

1.      Complete your grounding, centering, and shielding exercises

2.      Gather:      3              lodestone

                      1 tbsp         mint leaves

                      1 tbsp         mistletoe

                      1 tbsp         clover

                      1              small orange or yellow bag

3.      Cleanse and empower your ingredients

4.      Place the ingredients in the bag

5.      Hang the bag in a prominent place in the business

6.      Shake the bag each day to release the aroma and attract customers

## *Business Attracting Powder*

1.　Complete your grounding, centering, and shielding exercises

2.　Cleanse and empower your ingredients

3.　Gather:　　3 tbsp　　　finely powdered Irish moss

　　　　　　　　3 tbsp　　　finely powdered vetiver

　　　　　　　　3 tbsp　　　finely powdered clover

　　　　　　　　1　　　　　Small container with lid

4.　Blend the powders well

5.　Store in a clean, dry container with a tightly fitting lid

6.　Sprinkle a pinch of the powders around the business each day

## Business Bells

1.	Complete your grounding, centering, and shielding exercises

2.	Gather:    3          gold or tin bells

                3 drops    citronella oil

                3 drops    mint oil

                length    yellow or orange cord, string, or ribbon

3.	Cleanse and empower your ingredients

4.	Hold the bells in your hand and concentrate on the success you need

5.	Tie the bells together using your string, cord, or ribbon

6.	Anoint the bells and string, cord, or ribbon with the oils

7.	Hang the bells above or on the door to your business

8.	Recharge the bells with new oils each time you feel the need

9.	Each day when you arrive at your business say to the bells

Beautiful bells please use your song
bring me prosperity all day long

## Thriving Business Bowl

1.      Complete your grounding, centering, and shielding exercises

2.      Gather:        1                  gold or tin bowl

                       1 piece       skullcap

                       1 tsp          money oil of your choice

                       1                  length of yellow or green cord, yarn, or ribbon

3.      Cleanse and empower your ingredients

4.      Anoint the skullcap with the money oil until it is well moistened

5.      Wind the cord around the skullcap until it is completely covered leaving an end for a hanger

6.      Hang the skullcap above the door

7.      Mist the skullcap with new money oil at the beginning of each business week

Everyone who enters should feel the need to spend money

## Healing & Comfort Spells

Healing is probably the most universal of all alternative practices. Most alternative treatments are designed to treat a problem within the body, mind, or spirit. Many of the correspondences you have learned about address a specific ailment.

Healing is a little different because you will often be treating someone other than yourself through your craft. Just as belief in self is critical to successful spell craft, the belief of the person being treated is essential to success.

The suggested rituals, blends, and instructions on the following pages are just that suggestions based on the most effective steps we take to meet the needs of those who come to us seeking aide. As long as your intent is true and your and your partner's belief in your abilities is strong, these should work well for you. If you find yourself having difficulty with any instruction included, take time to ground, center yourself, and then meditate for a time on what you might do to adapt the inclusions so that they are better suited to your personal energies & abilities. The correspondences charts throughout this book might assist you in adapting the spell craft to meet your needs.

# *Magic Witches Ladder for Comfort and Blessing*

A witch's ladder is an excellent gift for a sick friend or loved one. It brings comfort and positive energy from your heart to the body of your friend.

1.    Complete your grounding, centering, and shielding exercises

2.    Obtain a long length of blue cord or ribbon

3.    Select 7 symbols to hang from it.

      These symbols must be meaningful to you and your friend.

      They should represent comfort, protection, and healing. Common ideas include

      ➢    grey feathers for protection during sleep

      ➢    sprigs of healing herbs

      ➢    garlic for healing and protection

      ➢    small talismans that are meaningful to you and your friend

      ➢    charms

      ➢    healing crystals and stones

4.    Cleanse and empower your ingredients

5.    Tie the symbols at equal distances along the cord imbuing each knot with comfort, energy, and positive thoughts.

# The Golden Cord Spell for Healing

You should begin this spell on a Monday

1.    Complete your grounding, centering, and shielding exercises

2.    Obtain a photograph or item of the sick person

3.    Select a thin yellow ribbon, rope, or hemp cord

4.    Cleanse and empower your ingredients

5     Hold the cord over the item and say;

"With knot of one, my spell's begun

     tie the 1st knot

"With knot of two my word is true,

     tie the 2nd knot

With knot of three, I bring healing to thee,

     tie the 3rd knot

By knot of four, you're better than before,

     tie the 4th knot

By knot of five you are no longer six,

     tie the 5th knot

By knot of six this spell's alive,

     tie the 6th knot

Seventh knot sealed, you are healed"

tie the 7th knot

"So mote it be"

6.   Give the string to the sick person to hang above their bed

## Quick Candle Healing Spell

1.   Complete your grounding, centering, and shielding exercises

2.   Gather a blue candle and a pin

3.   Cleanse and empower your ingredients

4.   Anoint the candle with the aromatic oils best designed to suit your purpose.

     You can gain ideas on the appropriate oils from the section title Herb & Oil Blends

5.   Use the pin to inscribe the name of the sick person on the candle

     Write from base to top

6.   Put the pin through the base of the candle

7.   Light the candle

8.   Allow the candle to burn until it puts itself out

# Worry Jar Spell

We all have worries, anxieties, and stress in our lives. When they begin to become so large that they interfere with the joy, happiness, and love in your life, you need to create a worry jar.

1. Complete your grounding, centering, and shielding exercises

2. Sterilize a jar or container with a tight fitting lid

3. Write the problems that are weighing you down on a slip of paper

4. Pass the paper through the 4 elements
   Pass the paper through the smoke of a candle
   Wave the paper through the air over the jar
   Sprinkle a few drops of water onto the paper
   Sprinkle the paper with a small amount of dirt of dirt

5. As you pass the paper through the elements, say

   Into this vessel secured up tight
   I place my anxieties that they might
   Find their right level within my life
   Be only acknowledged when I say it's right.
   I swear that I will not give thought to my woe
   Until such time to this vessel I go
   And take off the lid and grieve, for I know
   That unless the lid's missing, trapped is my foe.
   It may not escape into my daily way
   And trouble my thinking during the day.
   Some time in the future when I feel I may
   Dispose of this vessel with no debt to pay.

6. Place the jar on a windowsill that receives moonlight each night

7. Each time the problem sneaks into your mind, think of the jar.

8. You will find that soon, you will stop thinking about the problem.

9. When the problem is resolved, remove the slip and bury or burn it, giving thanks to the Lady.


## *Healing Vase Spell*

This vase should be given to the person in need of healing. If the problem is emotional, you can use the vase to help bring healing energies into the home.

1. Complete your grounding, centering, and shielding exercises

2. Gather           clear glass vase

                        blue and clear florist marbles

3. Cleanse the vase and water in cold spring water

4. Allow the vase and marbles to dry in the sun

5. Begin placing the marbles in the vase while saying

      Balls of blue Healing true

      Balls of clear Cleansing here


6. Use as a center piece or place in a prominent place.

# Magic Egyptian Knot Amulet

1. Complete your grounding, centering, and shielding exercises

2. Gather           a length of red string, ribbon, or embroidery floss

        1 tbsp      sea salt

        ½ cup      water

                  incense of your choice

        1 cup      melted candle wax

3. Cleanse and empower your ingredients

4. Knot or braid the red string into a bracelet while visualizing your need.

5. Knot the bracelet seven times. With each knot, say the seven names of the Goddess.

   - Isis
   - Astarte
   - Diana
   - Hecate
   - Demetere
   - Kali
   - Inanna

6. Bless the bracelet with Air by passing it through the Incense three times.

7. Bless it with Fire by passing it over the Candle three times.

8. Bless it with Water by sprinkling it with three drops of water

9. Bless it with Earth by passing it over the salt bowl three times.

10. Bless it with Life by blowing across it three times.

11. Tie the bracelet around your wrist with a square knot.

12. Say, "With this, the Lord and Lady shall shine light on shadows cast and keep me from harm's way, let this be done! So mote it be!"

## Spell to Create and Amulet for Well-Being

1. Place a piece of

    ➢ amber

    ➢ fresh mint

    ➢ slice of orange rind

    ➢ apple peel

    in a container.

2. Envision the bundle filled with a greenish white light while saying

    Keep sickness at bay, bring health each day!

    Keep sickness at bay, bring health each day!

    Keep sickness at bay, bring health each day!

3. Carry the bundle with you as often as possible.

# Healing Magnets

Magnets are used to draw out the non-physical cause of the pain.

1.     Complete your grounding, centering, and shielding exercises

2.     Gather     5     magnets (Lodestones)

               1     blue candle

3.     Cleanse and empower your ingredients

4.     Light the candle

5.     Place the magnets in a circle around the candle

6.     Burn the candle for 15 minutes a day

7.     After you blow out the candle, gather 4 of your magnets

8.     Rub the affected area with one of the magnets

9.     Place one of the magnets under your pillow while you sleep

10.    Add one of the magnets to your bath water

11.    Carry the last magnet with you at all times

12.    Repeat these steps each day until the pain has gone

# *Spell to Increase Health and Vitality*

1. Complete your grounding, centering, and shielding exercises

2. Locate a piece of Quartz Crystal that appeals to you

3. Wash the quartz in warm, soapy water

4. Rinse the quartz with fresh water

5. Hold the crystal in both hands.

6. Close your eyes and imagine being bathed in white light.

7. Visualize the area of your illness and point the crystal to that site.

8. Imagine a stream of light flowing from the crystal and bathing the area in its pure rays.

9. Place your crystal under your pillow while you sleep.

10. Repeat these steps each day until you feel better

# Spell for Healing Someone in Your Family

1.   Complete your grounding, centering, and shielding exercises

2,   Cut a Piece of Paper approximately 9x9

3.   Fold to create a pouch or envelope

4.   Label the envelope

    ➢   health

    ➢   Recipients Name

5.   Cleanse and empower your ingredients

6.   Add the appropriate herb or oil blend for the ailment you are trying to cure

7.   Say   I charge these herbs to aid my spell,
            that _____ (name of person) will be well,
            That by free will that can be blessed,
            with total health and happiness,
            I ask the Goddess to hear my call,
            that it may be correct and for the good of all

8.   Using your candle, set the envelope on fire.

9.   Place the envelope on a metal plate

10.   Focus on the smoke and visualize the energy blowing with the smoke toward those in need.

11.   Allow the envelope to burn

# Healthy Family Spell

This is a nice spell to protect you family from common illnesses, especially during cold and flu season.

1.  Complete your grounding, centering, and shielding exercises

2.  Gather:  1  wooden spoon
            1  bowl or dish
            1  3x3 square of muslin cloth

    Choose a color that represents peace and healing to you and your family.

    If you are not sure, you could choose white or blue

    Length of Red Ribbon, String, or Cord

3.  Add the herb blend of your choice.  If you are unsure which blend to use to achieve the best results, refer to the section regarding Herb & Oil Correspondences

4.  Cleanse and empower your ingredients

5.  Use the wooden spoon to blend the herbs in a bowl

6.  Say   I conjure thee to be a protection,
          I invoke the Magic of old,
          To keep my family healthy and well,
          So mote it be.

7.  Place the mixture onto the square of cloth

8.  Close the sides and tie with the red ribbon, leave a loop at the top

9.  Hang the healing pouch in a place that can benefit each member of the family.

10. Shake the pouch every day to release the scents within into the air

# Irish Healing Water

The Irish are known for having skills at creating energizing blends for healing, luck, and a positive life. Irish Healing Waters are one of the best known and effective healing agents.

These steps are best completed on a Wednesday

1.      Complete your grounding, centering, and shielding exercises

2.      Gather      2 cup       distilled water

                    ½ cup       lavender

                    ½ cup       violet

                    ½ cup       rosemary

3.      Cleanse and empower your ingredients

4.      Place all ingredients in a sterile iron pot

5.      Bring to a boil

6.      Reduce heat and simmer 30-45 minutes

7.      You should have a richly colored aromatic blend

8.      Strain the herbs from the water

9.      Pour the water into a clean jar with a tight lid

10.     Place the jar in sunlight for an entire day to absorb the radiant energies of the sun.

11.     Occasionally look at the jar and add your own energies to it.

12.     Just before sundown get the jar and hold it firmly between your hands Just below your naval.

13. Feel your desire to be well filling the jar and with your minds eye see it glowing brightly as the sun.

14. Say these words until you have filled the jar with as much energy as it will hold.

    By the herb and by the sun
    Wellness and I are now as one
    Strengthening energies now are merged.
    Baneful energies now be purged

15. Apply a few drops of the healing waters to the area where you suffer from illness or unhappiness.

    If you are not certain where the source of your discomfort is located, add ¼ cup to your bathwater each night.

16. Repeat the application daily until you feel better.


## *Depression Relief Spell*

1. Complete your grounding, centering, and shielding exercises

2. Gather

    | | | |
    |---|---|---|
    | 1 | white candle |
    | 1 | black marker |
    | 1 | kunzite or blue agate |
    | 1 tsp | lemon balm |
    | 3 drops | lemon oil |
    | 1 | blue Muslin Cloth Pouch |

3. Cleanse and empower your ingredients

4. Use the marker to color the candle black

This symbolizes the depression that surrounds you

5.   Light the candle

6.   Say   Flame cut through depression, deep
            Melt it down & make it weep
            Grant me power to re-emerge
            from its grip, I leap & surge

7.   Watch the candle burn until white wax appears at the flame.

8.   Rub a bit of lemon oil into the stone

9.   Say   Kunzite/agate, stone of mellow hue
            dissolve the depression, I beg of you
            Take its power & transform its strength
            Into positive energy I can use at length

10.  Lightly rub the stone against your temples & your heart

11.  Place the stone in front of the candle

12.  Sprinkle the stone with lemon balm

13.  Let the candle burn completely

14.  Place the stone & remaining herbs in the cloth pouch

15.  Carry the stone with you

# Healing Candle Blends

As you become more adept at formulating your own spell craft and gain a deeper understanding of the properties of different herbs and oils you will want to formulate custom blends that work well for you. These recipes are some of the most effective blends for the most common requests we receive from people seeking aide.

## Calming Scented Candle

| ½ tsp | adder's tongue |
|---|---|
| 9 drops | bay oil |
| 9 drops | chamomile oil |
| 9 drops | colorant – blue |
| 1 cup | candle wax base |

## Anti-Anxiety Daytime Scented Candle

| 6 drops | cedar oil |
|---|---|
| 6 drops | chamomile oil |
| 6 drops | cypress oil |
| 6 drops | lemon oil |
| 9 drops | colorant – blue |
| 1 cup | candle wax base |

### Anti-Anxiety Nighttime Scented Candle

| 9 drops | chamomile oil |
| 9 drops | cypress oil |
| 9 drops | lavender oil |
| 9 drops | valerian oil |
| 9 drops | colorant – blue |
| 1 cup | candle wax base |

### Memory Enhancing Scented Candle

| 6 drops | adder's tongue    oil |
| 6 drops | bay oil |
| 6 drops | clove oil |
| 6 drops | peppermint oil |
| 6 drops | rosemary oil |
| 9 drops | colorant – yellow |
| 1 cup | candle wax base |

### Stress Relief Scented Candle

| | |
|---|---|
| 1 tbsp | dried calamus |
| 1 tbsp | chamomile oil |
| 9 drops | colorant – blue |
| 1 cup | candle wax base |

### Insomnia Relief Scented Candle

| | |
|---|---|
| 1 ½ tbsp | scotch broom |
| 1 ½ tbsp | calamus |
| 9 drops | valerian oil |
| 9 drops | colorant – blue |
| 1 cup | candle wax base |

### Nightmare Relief Scented Candle

| | |
|---|---|
| 9 drops | cedar oil or 2 tbsp finely chipped cedar |
| 1 ½ tbsp | lavender leaves |
| 9 drops | valerian oil |
| 9 drops | colorant – blue |
| 1 cup | candle wax base |

## Headache Relief Candle

1 cup      candle wax base

1 tsp      bay

1 tsp      feverfew

1 tsp      lemon balm

1 tsp      betony

# Healing Herb and Oil Blends

These are some of the most effective herb & oil blends we use for the most common requests from people who seek aide. You can use these herbs & oils in poppets, dream pillows, candles, mojo bags, simmers, sprays, and sachets. You can also incorporate the blends into spells of your own design for additional powers.

There are many decent guides on herb and oil blends similar to my **Compendium of Beneficial Herbs & Oils.** As you advance in the craft, you will wish to obtain a guide of expanded herbs & oils, their properties, side effects, and use from a reputable source. The expanded guides will help you in creating your own spell craft and remedies.

## ADD, Hyperactivity, Loss of Focus Blend

½ tsp        adder's tongue

6 drops      bay oil

6 drops      chamomile oil

## Anti-Anxiety Daytime Blend

8 drops      cedar oil

8 drops      chamomile oil

8 drops      cypress oil

8 drops      lemon oil

## Anti-Anxiety Nighttime Blend

6 drops      chamomile oil

6 drops      cypress oil

6 drops      lavender oil

6 drops      valerian oil

## Memory Enhancing Blend

6 drops      adder's tongue oil

6 drops      bay oil

6 drops      clove oil

6 drops      peppermint oil

6 drops      rosemary oil

## Stress Reduction Blend

8 drops      cedar oil

8 drops      cypress oil

8 drops      sandalwood oil

## Cold & Flu Fighting Aromatic Blend

1 tbsp        clove oil

1 tbsp        fennel

1 tbsp        lemon oil

## Insomnia Relief Blend

8 drops      lavender oil

8 drops      chamomile oil

8 drops      ylang-ylang

## Wart Remover – 7 day treatment

2 tbsp        basil leaves

2 tbsp        dandelion flower juice

Blend well

Apply a thin coat to wart

Allow to dry

Repeat every 2 hours as needed until wart falls off

## Nightmare Relief

| 1 tsp | bay leaves |
|---|---|
| 1 tsp | anise seed |
| 4 drops | lavender oil |
| 4 drops | chamomile oil |

## Pain Relief Aromatic Blend

| 1 tsp | bay |
|---|---|
| 1 tsp | feverfew |
| 1 tsp | lemon balm |
| 1 tsp | betony |

# CHAPTER 16

## Cleansing & Protection Spells

Cleansings are important to repel negative energies and to help open the way to positive energies & blessings. I cleanse my house, car, and person on a regular basis to allow positive energies & blessings easier access and to help the beneficial spells work better.

### *Broom Purification*

1.   Complete your grounding, centering, and shielding exercises

2.   Take a branch from any tree

3.   Thank the tree for its gift

4.   Leave a coin or semi-precious stone at its base in payment

5.   Select several brightly colored flowers on long stalks.

6.   Tie the flowers to the branch to create a broom

7.   Sweep the floor in every room of the house

8.   Visualize the flowers of the broom absorbing negativity as you work.

9.   Leave the broom at the crossroads

10.   Repeat the first day of each month

## Self-Cleansing Bath

This ritual bath is designed to cleanse your mind, body, & spirit of negativity.

1.      Cleanse and empower your ingredients

2.      Gather      1              white candle anointed or made with

                    3 drops       pine oil

                    3 drops       rosemary oil

                    3 drops       eucalyptus oil

                    2 tbsp        sea salt

3.      Brew         1 tbsp        hyssop

                    1 tbsp        sage          into a strong tea

4.      Draw a hot bath

5.      Pour the tea into the bathwater

6.      Add the sea salt to the water

7.      Stir the water with your left hand to dissolve the salts and blend the tea

8.      Place the candle so that you can see the light shining on you when you get into the tub

9.      Light the candle

10.     Immerse yourself in the water

11.     Complete your grounding, centering, and shielding exercises while soaking in the bath

12.     Drain the water but do not rinse off the bath

## *Cleansing & Purification Smoke*

This purification will cleanse your body of any negative accumulations while cleansing the air in the room.

1.    Complete your grounding, centering, and shielding exercises

2.    Gather        1 each        pine, rosemary, cinnamon, and thyme incense
                                   sticks bound together with a white cord

      or             1             white candle anointed or made with
                                   3 drops      pine oil
                                   3 drops      rosemary oil
                                   3 drops      cinnamon
                                   2 tbsp       thyme

3.    Cleanse and empower your ingredients

4.    Light the bound incense stick bundle or the candle

5.    Pass the smoke around your body

6.    Breath deeply to help the aromatics enter inside your body

6.    Picture the smoke surrounding your body and passing through every fiber of your being

7.    Envision the negativity leaving you as the aromatic smoke forces negativity out of your body and cleanses it from the skin

8.    When you feel cleansed, allow the incense sticks or candle to burn completely cleansing the air in the room

9.    You may carry the sticks or candle around the house waving the aromatic smoke into each corner and place to help speed the cleansing process and inhibit any latent negativity in the home from attaching to your newly cleansed body

## Home Purification Wash

This purification will cleanse your home of any negative accumulations

1. Complete your grounding, centering, and shielding exercises

2. Gather
   | | |
   |---|---|
   | 7 drops | pine oil |
   | 7 drops | juniper oil |
   | 7 drops | cedar oil |
   | 7 drops | rosemary oil |
   | 7 drops | eucalyptus oil |
   | 1 quart | spring water |

3. Cleanse and empower your ingredients

4. Mix oils and water – these will separate so make certain you blend well

5. Lightly mist the floor, walls, fabric, & other areas of your home

6. Repeat at least once a week

## Home Purification Powder

This purification will cleanse your home of any negative accumulations

1.      Complete your grounding, centering, and shielding exercises

2.      Gather

| | |
|---|---|
| 1 cup | salt |
| 1 cup | baking soda |
| 1 tbsp | powdered juniper needles |
| 1 tbsp | powdered rosemary |
| 1 tbsp | powdered pine needles |
| 1 tbsp | powdered cedar |

3.      Cleanse and empower your ingredients

4.      Blend ingredients

5.      Sprinkle a small amount on the floors of each room making certain you reach under furniture and in the corners

6.      Allow to sit for at least 30 minutes

7.      Sweep with a broom or sweeper

8.      Discard the sweepings OUTSIDE the home, burying them in the farthest corner of your yard if possible

.

## Hex Removing Bath

This ritual bath is designed to cleanse your mind, body, & spirit of negativity.

1. Complete your grounding, centering, and shielding exercises

2. Gather 1 Red Candle

   7 drops linden oil

   3 tbsp nutmeg

   3 tbsp sea salt

3. Cleanse and empower your ingredients

4. Draw a hot bath

5. Sprinkle the oils, salts, & herbs in your bath water

6. Stir the water with your left hand to dissolve the salts and blend the oils & herbs

7. Place the candle so that you can see the light shining on you when you get into the tub

8. Light the candle

9. Immerse yourself in the water

10. Complete your grounding, centering, and shielding exercises while soaking in the bath

11. Drain the water but do not rinse off the bath

## Hex Breaking Smoke

1. Complete your grounding, centering, and shielding exercises

2. Gather     1 each     betony, vetiver, verbena, agrimony incense sticks bound together with a white cord

   or

   1     white candle anointed or made with

   3 drops     betony

   3 drops     vertiver

   3 drops     verbena

   3 drops     agrimony

3. Cleanse and empower your ingredients

4. Light the bound incense stick bundle or the candle

5. Pass the smoke around your body

6. Breath deeply to help the aromatics enter inside your body

6. Picture the smoke surrounding your body and passing through every fiber of your being

7. Envision the hex leaving you as the aromatic smoke forces negativity out of your body and cleanses it from the skin

8. When you feel cleansed, allow the incense sticks or candle to burn completely cleansing the air in the room of any residual effects

9. You may carry the sticks or candle around the house waving the aromatic smoke into each corner and place to help speed the removal process and inhibit any latent negativity in the home from attaching to your newly cleansed body

## Home Hex Removal Wash

This purification will cleanse your home of any negative accumulations and break a hex that has been cast against you or your household

1.      Complete your grounding, centering, and shielding exercises

2.      Gather        7 drops        holly thistle oil

                        7 drops        juniper oil

                        7 drops        rosemary oil

                        7 drops        eucalyptus oil

                        7 drops        pennyroyal oil

                        1 quart        spring water

3.      Cleanse and empower your ingredients

4.      Mix oils and water – these will separate so make certain you blend well

5.      Lightly mist the floor, walls, fabric, & other areas of your home

6.      Repeat any time you feel that you are in a negative place or a hex has been cast against you or your household

## *Home Purification Powder*

This purification will cleanse your home of any negative accumulations

1.  Complete your grounding, centering, and shielding exercises

2.  Gather

|         |                        |
|---------|------------------------|
| 1 cup   | salt                   |
| 1 cup   | baking soda            |
| 1 tbsp  | powdered holly thistle |
| 1 tbsp  | powdered nettle        |
| 1 tbsp  | powdered pennyroyal    |

3.  Cleanse and empower your ingredients

4.  Blend ingredients

5.  Sprinkle a small amount on the floors of each room making certain you reach under furniture and in the corners

6.  Allow to sit for at least 30 minutes

7.  Sweep with a broom or sweeper

8.  Discard the sweepings OUTSIDE the home, burying them in the farthest corner of your yard if possible

## *Reversal Poppet*

1. Complete your grounding, centering, and shielding exercises

2. Cleanse and empower your ingredients

3. Create a white poppet

4. Stuff the poppet with cayenne pepper, coffee grounds, and violets

5. Inscribe your name on a white candle anointed with or created with your preferred herb & oil blend

6. Visualize the hex you believe was cast against you

7. Feel the power the hex has had in your life

8. Take a handful of holly thistle and sprinkle it over the poppet

9. Visualize the hex being broken

10. Lay the poppet in front of your candle

11. Allow the candle to burn down completely

12. Place a piece of iron or copper in the poppet's hand

13. Bury the poppet off your property

14. If you cannot discard the poppet, lock it along with the piece of copper or iron in a place where it cannot do any harm

## *Hex Reflecting & Protecting Amulet*

1.  Complete your grounding, centering, and shielding exercises

2.  Gather      1        small red flannel bag

            1        piece of clear quartz

            1        piece of iron or brass

            pinch    cayenne pepper

            6 drops  fresh brewed coffee

            3 drops  musk oil

            3 drops  violet oil

3.  Cleanse and empower your ingredients

4.  Place the piece of quartz & metal inside your bag

5.  Sprinkle the herbs & oils over your cleansed pieces of quartz & metal

6.  Seal the bag tightly

7.  Carry the bag with you to help absorb the power of the curse, reflect the curse back to the sender, and remove the curse from you

## Protection Incense or Candle Blend

1.   Complete your grounding, centering, and shielding exercises

2.   Gather      1 each      clove, juniper, and thistle incense sticks bound
                              together with a red cord

                              or

              1              white candle anointed or made with

                      3 drops      clove oil

                      1 tsp        crushed juniper berries

                      1 tsp        curry powder

                      1 tsp        thistle

3.   Cleanse and empower your ingredients

4.   Light the bound incense stick bundle or the candle

5.   Pass the smoke around your body

6.   Breath deeply to help the aromatics enter inside your body

6.   Picture the smoke surrounding your body and passing through every fiber
     of your being

7.   Envision the aromatic smoke spreading protection to the farthest reaches
     of your body

8.   Allow the incense sticks or candle to burn completely cleansing the air in
     the room of any residual effects

9.   You may carry the sticks or candle around the house waving the aromatic
     smoke into each corner and place to help speed the protection process
     and repel any new negativity trying to enter

## *Home Protection Mist*

This mist will bar evil and negativity from entering your home

1. Complete your grounding, centering, and shielding exercises

2. Gather      7 drops      dogwood oil

                        7 drops      lemon oil

                        7 drops      musk oil

                        7 drops      rose geranium oil

                        1 quart      spring water

3. Cleanse and empower your ingredients

4. Mix oils and water – these will separate so make certain you blend well

5. Lightly mist the openings of your home, doorknobs, walls, & floors

6. Repeat daily or weekly as your needs demand

## *Home Protection Powder*

This powder will help to repel negativity and evil from the home

1.      Complete your grounding, centering, and shielding exercises

2.      Gather

|         |                         |
|---------|-------------------------|
| 4 tbsp  | salt                    |
| 1 tbsp  | powdered elder berries  |
| 1 tbsp  | powdered cumin          |
| 1 tbsp  | powdered barley         |
| 1 tbsp  | powdered morning glory  |

3.      Cleanse and empower your ingredients

4.      Blend ingredients

5.      Sprinkle a small amount in the corners of each room to protect from negativity

6.      Repeat weekly

## Home Protecting Amulet

1.      Complete your grounding, centering, and shielding exercises

2.      Gather

| | | |
|---|---|---|
| 1 | small red flannel bag |
| 1 | quartz |
| 1 | piece brass |
| 3 | dill seeds |
| 3 | flax seeds |
| 1 tsp | marjoram |
| 1 tsp | spearmint |

3.      Cleanse and empower your ingredients

4.      Place the piece of seeds, quartz, & brass inside your bag

5.      Sprinkle the herbs over your cleansed seeds, quartz, & metal

6.      Seal the bag tightly

7.      Hang the bag near the main entry of the home or in the place where the family gathers

## Home Protection Wreath or Door Sash

1.  Complete your grounding, centering, and shielding exercises

2.  Gather     1          length of white cord

                    1          length of red cord

                    1          length of blackberry vine

                    1          length of st. john's root

                    1          length of sweet grass

3.  Cleanse and empower your ingredients

4.  Weave or braid all of the lengths together to form a wreath or sash that appeals to you

5.  Hang on or over the doorway to repel negativity & keep positive energies flowing

## Protectant Potpourri

1. Complete your grounding, centering, and shielding exercises

2. Gather     ½ cup     baking soda

   1     finely chopped comfrey root

   2 tbsp     coriander

   7 drops     patchouli

   1     cleansed & charged brass bowl

3. Cleanse and empower your ingredients

4. Place the baking soda in the bottom of the bowl

5. Mix the herbs & oils

6. Pour the herbs on top of the baking soda

5. Place in a well-used room of your home

6. Whenever the benefits seem to be fading, gently stir the mixture to release the scent into the air

7. Replace every 30 days as needed

## Protective candle

To dispel negativity, cleanse a space, and protect the inhabitants

| 1 cup | melted candle base |
|-------|--------------------|
| 1 tsp | basil |
| 1 tsp | bay |
| 1 tsp | cloves |
| 1 tsp | rosemary |

## Personal Protection Oil for Men

This mist will bar evil, negativity, and harm from touching you

1. Complete your grounding, centering, and shielding exercises
2. Gather
   - 3 drops — clove oil
   - 3 drops — cypress oil
   - 3 drops — musk oil
   - 4 tbsp — carrier oil such as jojoba or coconut
3. Cleanse and empower your ingredients
4. Mix oils until well blended
5. Place in a clean, airtight container
6. Anoint yourself with a few drops of the oil twice each day

## *Personal Protection Spray for Women*

This mist will bar evil, negativity, and harm from touching you

1.  Complete your grounding, centering, and shielding exercises

2.  Gather     3 drops     lily oil

                      3 drops     lilac oil

                      3 drops     frangipani oil

                      4 tbsp     carrier oil such as jojoba or coconut

3.  Cleanse and empower your ingredients

4.  Mix oils until well blended

5.  Place in a clean, airtight container

6.  Anoint yourself with a few drops of the oil twice each day

## Personal Protection Amulet Bag

This bag will help to repel negativity and evil and protect you from harm

1.  Complete your grounding, centering, and shielding exercises

2.  Gather

    | 1 small | red bag |
    |---------|---------|
    | 1 tsp | clove |
    | 1 tsp | lilac |
    | 1 tsp | bruised dill |
    | 1 tsp | rue |
    | 3 drops | musk oil |
    | 3 drops | cypress oil |

3.  Cleanse and empower your ingredients

4.  Place ingredients in bag

5.  Shake well

6.  Tie the bag closed

7.  Carry with you shaking the bag to release the aroma whenever you feel especially vulnerable

## *Personal Protecting Amulet*

1.  Complete your grounding, centering, and shielding exercises

2.  Gather      1            small red flannel bag

                   1            opal

                   1            piece brass

                   1 tsp        chamomile

                   1 tsp        cinnamon

                   1 tsp        clover

                   1 tsp        rosemary

3.  Cleanse and empower your ingredients

4.  Place the piece of opal & brass inside your bag

5.  Sprinkle the herbs over your cleansed opal & brass

6.  Seal the bag tightly

7.  Carry the bag with you at all times, sleep with it under your pillow at night

## *Traveler's Protective Charm*

1. Complete your grounding, centering, and shielding exercises

2. Gather

| | | |
|---|---|---|
| 1 | small blue flannel bag |
| 1 | malachite stone |
| 1 | piece brass |
| 1 tsp | chopped comfrey root |
| 1 tsp | feverfew |
| 1 tsp | mint |
| 1 tsp | morning glory |

3. Cleanse and empower your ingredients

4. Place the piece of malachite & brass inside your bag

5. Sprinkle the herbs over your cleansed malachite & brass

6. Seal the bag tightly

7. Place the bag in your car to aid in safe travel or carry with you when traveling in another vehicle

# Protective & Cleansing Herb & Oil Blends

These are some of the most effective herb & oil blends we use for the most common requests from people who seek aide. You can use these herbs & oils in poppets, dream pillows, candles, mojo bags, simmers, sprays, and sachets. You can also incorporate the blends into spells of your own design for additional powers.

There are many decent guides on herb and oil blends similar to my **Compendium of Beneficial Herbs & Oils.** As you advance in the craft, you will wish to obtain a guide of expanded herbs & oils, their properties, side effects, and use from a reputable source. The expanded guides will help you in creating your own spell craft and remedies.

## Prosperity, Happiness & Protection Blend

| | |
|---|---|
| 1 tbsp | allspice |
| 1 tbsp | almond |
| 1 tbsp | cinnamon |
| 3 drops | lime juice |

## Home & Person Protection Blend

| | |
|---|---|
| 1 tsp | basil |
| 1 tsp | bay |
| 1 tsp | cloves |
| 1 tsp | bergamot |

## Potpourri to Draw Good Luck & Protect from Negative Energies

| | |
|---|---|
| 3 tbsp | juniper berries |
| 3 tbsp | basil |
| 3 tbsp | frankincense |
| 3 tbsp | crushed dill seeds |
| 3 tbsp | crushed clove |
| 3 tbsp | shredded bay leaves |

Blend herbs well and place in small bowls or jars around them home to draw good luck and protect from negative energies


## Space Protection & Purification Blend

| | |
|---|---|
| 5 drops | basil oil |
| 5 drops | bay oil |
| 5 drops | sage oil |
| 5 drops | eucalyptus oil |
| 5 drops | lavender oil |
| 2 tbsp | lemon juice |

## Negativity Repelling Blend

Use daily to change your luck, enhance personal protection from negativity, injury, and harm and to break hexes

| 1 tsp | basil |
| 1 tsp | bay |
| 1 tsp | chamomile |
| 1 tsp | rosemary |

## Traveler's Protection Blend

| 1 tbsp | bladder wrack |
| 1 tbsp | feverfew |
| 1 tbsp | peppermint |

# CHAPTER 17

## Anger & Friendship Spells

Anger can taint every aspect of your life. Whether the anger comes from inside you or is directed at you, banishing anger is one of the most proactive steps you can take to bring joy and blessings to your life.

At times, it is possible to turn an angry person into a friend so we have combined these two groupings into one spell section

Friendship, like anything, is dependent on many factors. You can help to channel the natural world to increase your ability to attract life long friends, but you must also remove anger from your heart, cleanse your soul, and accept who you are to attract friends.

A pure heart & mind combined with a strong belief & love for yourself is the first, and most important, ingredient in friendship work. In fact, belief in your ability to channel the natural world to achieve your goals is the most important ingredient to success in any endeavor.

The suggested rituals, blends, and instructions on the following pages are just that suggestions based on the most effective steps we take to meet the needs of those who come to us seeking aide. As long as your intent is true and your belief in yourself is strong, these should work well for you. If you find yourself having difficulty with any instruction included, take time to ground, center yourself, and then meditate for a time on what you might do to adapt the inclusions so that they are better suited to your personal energies & abilities. The correspondences charts throughout this book might assist you in adapting the spell craft to meet your needs.

### *Strife Reducing Plant*

A live valerian plant in the home will help keep balance and harmony

### *Anti-Strife Powder*

This powder will help to repel negativity and evil from the home

1.  Complete your grounding, centering, and shielding exercises

2.  Gather     4 tbsp     salt

    1 tbsp     powdered lavender

    1 tbsp     powdered peach

    1 tbsp     powdered valerian

3.  Cleanse and empower your ingredients

4.  Blend ingredients

5.  Sprinkle a small amount in the corners of each room to dispel anger and encourage tranquility & communications

6.  Repeat weekly

## Incense or Candle to Bring Peace & Harmony

This incense will help stop gossip, make those who are angry stop to listen to the other party and restore peace, harmony, & togetherness to the home

1. Complete your grounding, centering, and shielding exercises

2. Gather     1 each     clove, lavender, valerian incense sticks bound together with a red cord

   or

   1     blue candle anointed or made with

       3 drops     clove oil

       3 drops     lavender oil

       3 drops     valerian

3. Cleanse and empower your ingredients

4. Light the bound incense stick bundle or the candle

5. Pass the smoke around your body

6. Breath deeply to help the aromatics enter inside your body

6. Picture the smoke surrounding your body and passing through every fiber of your being

7. Envision the aromatic smoke spreading protection to the farthest reaches of your body

8. Carry the sticks or candle around the house waving the aromatic smoke into each corner and place to help speed the removal of negativity and imbue the air with energies that promote peace, harmony, & happiness

## *Home Protection Mist*

This mist will help to remove negative energies and calm fighting parties to aid in restoring peace, harmony, & happiness to the home

1.    Complete your grounding, centering, and shielding exercises

2.    Gather     7 drops     balsam oil

                  7 drops     basil oil

                  7 drops     lilac oil

                  7 drops     coltsfoot oil

                  1 quart     spring water

3.    Cleanse and empower your ingredients

4.    Mix oils and water – these will separate so make certain you blend well

5.    Lightly mist the openings of your home, doorknobs, walls, & floors

6.    Repeat daily or weekly as your needs demand

## Strife Amulet

1. Complete your grounding, centering, and shielding exercises

2. Gather

| | | |
|---|---|---|
| 1 | small blue flannel bag |
| 1 | citrine |
| 1 | piece iron |
| 1 | leaf of iron weed |
| 1 | bitter aloe leaf |
| 1 tsp | bruised basil |
| 1 tsp | bruised gardenia |

3. Cleanse and empower your ingredients

4. Place the iron weed, aloe leaf, piece of citrine and iron inside your bag

5. Sprinkle the herbs over your cleansed items

6. Seal the bag tightly

7. Hang the bag near the place where the family gathers or carry it with you to help sooth tensions, repel negativity, and encourage peaceful communication

## Binding & Dispelling Poppet or Doll

1.    Complete your grounding, centering, and shielding exercises

2.    Cleanse and empower your ingredients

3.    Create a poppet using blue

4.    Sew a small piece of iron inside the doll

5.    Add the beneficial herb or oil blend that suits your needs

6.    Add any personal item from the person you are trying to bind or whose behavior you wish to improve.  This could be a photograph, piece of writing, hair, nail clipping, or other item

7.    Obtain one black and one red candles

8.    Anoint the candles with the appropriate oil blend for your needs

9.    Set the doll between the candles

9.    Light the candles

10.   Meditate and think of the person whose behavior is harming you

11.   Say     With harm to none
              my will be done
              I hereby bind
              leave the bad behind
              Your words cannot hurt me
              your thoughts do not harm me
              your behavior cannot touch me

12.   Visualize the person unable to reach through the protective smoke

13.   Place the doll between the candles

14.   Bury the doll far from you and your home

## Amulet to Release Anger

1.    Complete your grounding, centering, and shielding exercises

2.    Obtain a piece of citrine that feels right in your hands

3.    Buy or obtain a length of iron wire

4.    Cleanse the citrine and wire

5.    Charge the citrine for at least 24 hours

6.    Bind the citrine in the iron banding leaving a tail end to attach the amulet to a necklace, bracelet, or as a hanging crystal

7.    Wear or carry the citrine with you at all times

8.    Whenever you feel anger, rub the citrine as you star into it releasing your angry feelings into the crystal

9.    Cleanse the citrine with salt and water after each day

10.   Energize the crystal each night

## Strife Removing Potpourri

1. Complete your grounding, centering, and shielding exercises

2. Gather       ½ cup      baking soda

                   1 tbsp      basil

                   1 tbsp      balsam

                   7 drops      cypress oil

                   1 tbsp      bruised flax seeds

                   1      cleansed & charged iron bowl

3. Cleanse and empower your ingredients

4. Place the baking soda in the bottom of the bowl

5. Mix the herbs & oils

6. Pour the herbs on top of the baking soda

5. Place in a well-used room of your home

6. Whenever the benefits seem to be fading, gently stir the mixture to release the scent into the air

7. Replace every 30 days as needed

## Fight Repelling Candle Blend

| | |
|---|---|
| 1 cup | melted candle base |
| 7 drops | blue colorant |
| 1 tsp | powdered clove |
| 1 tsp | finely ground valerian |
| 1 tsp | powdered lavender |

## Gossip & Strife Protection Oil

This mist will help calm negative behavior and promote positive actions in others

1. Complete your grounding, centering, and shielding exercises

2. Gather

   | | |
   |---|---|
   | 3 drops | gardenia oil |
   | ¼ tsp | cucumber juice |
   | 3 drops | lilac oil |
   | 4 tbsp | carrier oil such as jojoba or coconut |

3. Cleanse and empower your ingredients

4. Mix oils until well blended

5. Place in a clean, airtight container

6. Anoint yourself with a few drops of the oil twice each day

## Reconciliation Amulet

Trace your hand and write the person's name in the palm in your picture

Wrap it and tie it up around a piece of iron weed

"I open my hand and heart, so that anger may depart."

Carry the amulet with you whenever you see the person

## Forgiveness Spell

To forgive your own mistakes or those of others

1. Complete your grounding, centering, and shielding exercises

2. Gather    3 x 3         square of thin white paper or parchment

          1            pen charged with ink

          1            glass jar with a tight fitting lid

          ¼ cup        vinegar

3. Cleanse and empower your ingredients

4. Meditate on the wrong that has been done

5. Write the wrong on the parchment using the charged ink

6. Place the vinegar inside the jar

7. Immerse the paper in the vinegar

8. Seal the jar tightly to trap the wrong inside

9. Set the jar in the sunlight until the vinegar dissolves the wrong

10. Bury the jar away from your sight

### Amulet Bag to Attract Friendship

1.  Complete your grounding, centering, and shielding exercises

2.  Gather    1           length of gold or silver chain

            1           cleansed & charged turquoise

            3 drops     grape seed oil

            3 drops     sweet pea oil

            3 drops     passion flower oil

3.  Cleanse and empower your ingredients

4.  Anoint the stone with your oils

5.  Wear the stone on the chain each time you leave the house

6.  Cleanse, charge, & anoint your stone regularly


### Negativity Banishment & Friendship Attractant Knot Spell

1.  Complete your grounding, centering, and shielding exercises

2.  Gather    3 lengths of a silk, cord, or ribbon

            1       red

            1       blue

            1       white

approximately each 9-12 inches in length

3.  Cleanse and empower your ingredients

4. Braid the lengths of cord together until you have one long piece

5. Tie 9 knots in the braid while saying

Tie knot 1 while saying

> By knot of one, my spell's begun

Tie knot 2 while saying

> By knot of two, plenty of happy things to do

Tie knot 3 while saying

> By knot of three, friends & happiness comes to me

Tie knot 4 while saying

> By knot of four, friendship knocks at my door

Tie knot 5 while saying

> By knot of five, my emotions thrive

Tie knot 6 while saying

> By knot of six, this spell is fixed

Tie knot 7 while saying

> By knot of seven, happiness is given

Tie knot 8 while saying

> By knot of eight, peace is great

Tie knot 9 while saying

> By knot of nine, these things are mine

6.    Use the cord as a bracelet, carry the cord with you, or wear it as a necklace amulet cord

## Strife Incense or Candle Blend

This blend helps to sooth tempers, bring fighting people together and help to bring peace to the relationship during troubled times

| 1 cup | melted candle wax |
| 9 drops | colorant – blue |
| 1 ½ tsp herb or 9 drops oil | valerian |
| 1 ½ tsp herb or 9 drops oil | basil |
| 1 ½ tsp herb or 9 drops oil | lavender |
| 1 ½ tsp herb or 9 drops oil | ylang-ylang |

# Strife & Anger Herb & Oil Blends

These are some of the most effective herb & oil blends we use for the most common requests from people who seek aide. You can use these herbs & oils in poppets, dream pillows, candles, mojo bags, simmers, sprays, and sachets. You can also incorporate the blends into spells of your own design for additional powers.

There are many decent guides on herb and oil blends similar to my **Compendium of Beneficial Herbs & Oils.** As you advance in the craft, you will wish to obtain a guide of expanded herbs & oils, their properties, side effects, and use from a reputable source. The expanded guides will help you in creating your own spell craft and remedies

## Strife Blend

This blend helps sooth tempers, bring fighting people together and help to bring peace to the relationship during troubled times

10 drops oil  valerian

10 drops oil  basil

10 drops oil  lavender

10 drops oil  ylang-ylang

## Ended Relationship Blend

To help separate your emotions and get over the pain of an ended relationship

2 tbsp        basil leaves

1 tsp         camphor

1 tbsp        cayenne pepper

## *Friendship Oils*

Anoint the wrists, forearms, belly, & backs of knees with these oils daily to attract people to you and gain the opportunity to make them lifelong friends

1.     Complete your grounding, centering, and shielding exercises

2.     Gather      3 drops      grape seed oil

                     3 drops      sweet pea oil

                     3 drops      passion flower oil

                     4 tbsp       carrier oil such as jojoba or coconut

3.     Cleanse and empower your ingredients

4.     Mix oils until well blended

5.     Place in a clean, airtight container

6.     Anoint yourself with a few drops of the oil twice each day

# CHAPTER 18

## Spells to Draw Love

True and lasting love, like anything, is dependent on many factors. True love takes patience, dedication, and the ability to open yourself to the possibilities.

Through careful spell work, you can help to channel the natural world to increase your opportunity to find love, but you must also believe in yourself and your ability to BE loved.

Belief in self is the first, and most important, ingredient in love attraction work. In fact, belief in your ability to channel the natural world to achieve your goals is the most important ingredient to success in any endeavor.

The suggested rituals, blends, and instructions on the following pages are just that suggestions based on the most effective steps we take to meet the needs of those who come to us seeking aide. As long as your intent is true and your belief in yourself is strong, these should work well for you. If you find yourself having difficulty with any instruction included, take time to ground, center yourself, and then meditate for a time on what you might do to adapt the inclusions so that they are better suited to your personal energies & abilities. The correspondences charts throughout this book might assist you in adapting the spell craft to meet your needs.

## *Women's Love Oil Bottle*

This oil will aid a women in attracting the attention of a man.

1.      Complete your grounding, centering, and shielding exercises

2.      Cleanse and empower your ingredients

3.      Take a tall, thin bottle and add

   3 drops      gardenia oil

   3 drops      jasmine oil

   3 drops      sweet pea

   3 drops      ylang-ylang

4.      Mix

   2 tbsp       jojoba oil

   7 drops      red food coloring

5.      Fill jar to the top with red mixture

6.      Each day, shake the mixture well and apply one drop to your wrists, forearms, the back of the knees, and behind each ear

## Men's Love Oil Bottle

This oil will aid a man in attracting the attention of a woman.

1.      Complete your grounding, centering, and shielding exercises

2.      Cleanse and empower your ingredients

3.      Take a tall, thin bottle and add

    3 drops       civet oil

    3 drops       clove oil

    3 drops       bay pea

    3 drops       ylang-ylang

4.      Mix

    2 tbsp       jojoba oil

    7 drops       red food coloring

5.      Fill jar to the top with red mixture

6.      Each day, shake the mixture well and apply one drop to your wrists, forearms, the back of the knees, and behind each ear

## Love Drawing Herb Bag

This bag will attract new love or help to strengthen existing love

1.   Complete your grounding, centering, and shielding exercises

2.   Cleanse and empower your ingredients

3.   Gather        1 red bag

                   1 tsp   finely chopped sambul root

                   1 tsp   finely chopped mandrake root

                   1 tsp   finely chopped moss

                   1 tsp   finely chopped parsley

                   1 tsp   powdered white willow

4.   Stir the herbs well

5.   Seal the bag and carry it with you

6.   Shake the bag each morning and then open to inhale the aroma

## *Love Attractant Charm*

This charm helps attract the attention of others in a positive way and opens the door to finding a true and binding love.

1.  Complete your grounding, centering, and shielding exercises

2.  Gather    1    red flannel bag

                    1 tsp  catmint

                    1 tsp  basil

                    1 tsp  bay

                    1 tsp  marjoram

                    1       lodestone

3.  Cleanse and empower your ingredients

4.  Place all of the ingredients in the bag

5.  Shake the bag each morning

6.  Inhale the scents

7.  Carry with you to attract love

## Love Attraction Sachet

This amulet bag should be carried with you at all times to help you find the perfect love for you

1.      Complete your grounding, centering, and shielding exercises

2.      Gather      1            red flannel bag

                1 tsp        dill flowers

                1 tsp        geranium flowers

                1 tsp        rose petals

                1 tsp        vervain

                3 drops      ylang-ylang oil

3.      Cleanse and empower your ingredients

4.      Place the herbs inside the flannel bag

5.      Anoint with oil

6.      Shake the bag each morning and night to attract love

7.      Carry the bag with you at all times

## Love Locating Bath

This bath will help you attract the attention of the one that is meant to be with you. Use this bath each day before you leave your home. When you cross the path of the one that is meant to be with you, your energies will draw their attention.

1.    Complete your grounding, centering, and shielding exercises

2.    Brew a tea of       1 tsp        chamomile

                          1 tsp        marigold

                          1 tsp        hyacinth

                          1 tsp        passion flower

                          4 cups       spring water

3.    Cleanse and empower your ingredients

4.    Draw a hot bath

5.    Add the tea to the bathwater

6.    Soak the body and hair in the water for at least 30 minutes

7.    Do not rinse

## Love Attractant Amulet

This charm helps attract the attention of others in a positive way and opens the door to finding a true and binding love.

1.      Complete your grounding, centering, and shielding exercises

2.      Gather          1              rhyolite

                        1              chain of silver or gold

                        3 drops        frangipani

3.      Cleanse and empower your ingredients

4.      Anoint the stone with the oils

5.      Wear around the neck to draw love

6.      Refresh the oils each day until the one you want is yours

## Love Promoting Candle

1 cup         melted candle base

9 drops       red colorant

1             finely chopped aloe leaf

1 tsp         powdered coltsfoot

1 tsp         powdered coriander

6 drops       ylang-ylang

6 drops       coconut oil

# Love & Sex Herb & Oil Blends

These are some of the most effective herb & oil blends we use for the most common requests from people who seek aide.  You can use these herbs & oils in poppets, dream pillows, candles, mojo bags, simmers, sprays, and sachets.  You can also incorporate the blends into spells of your own design for additional powers.

There are many decent guides on herb and oil blends similar to my **Compendium of Beneficial Herbs & Oils.**  As you advance in the craft, you will wish to obtain a guide of expanded herbs & oils, their properties, side effects, and use from a reputable source.  The expanded guides will help you in creating your own spell craft and remedies

## Aphrodisiac Smoke

1 tbsp        damiana

## Love Attracting Blend

1 tsp        basil

1 tsp        calendula marigolds

1 tsp        chamomile

1 tsp        cloves

1 tsp        lavender

## Love Inspiring Blend

6 drops     clove oil

6 drops     ginger root

6 drops     jasmine oil

6 drops     ylang-ylang

# CHAPTER 19

## Herb Correspondences

| | |
|---|---|
| Acacia | Worn to aid meditation |
| | Develop psychic powers |
| | Divination |
| Agrimony | Burn to reverse & turn back spells |
| Ague Weed | Burn to stop hexes & crossings from getting to you |
| Allspice | Rub on the feet & chest to add strength to one's will power |
| | Brings prosperity, health & protection |
| Almond | Attract money, good fortune & wealth |
| | Added to money incenses & potions |
| Alfalfa | Bring good fortune in matters of money, business and good luck in gambling |
| | Keep sprigs in the home or as part of a mojo bag to keep poverty away & help you prosper |
| All Heal | Sprinkle in the room of the sick to cure illness |
| All Spice | Burned as an incense to attract money or luck |
| Allspice Berries | Good luck charms |
| | Draws fortune in business and gambling |
| | Worn on the person in a cloth bag to relieve mental stress |
| Almond | Used to anoint money & candles in prosperity rituals |
| | Used in money incense |
| Aloe | Hung over houses and doors to bring good luck |
| | Prevents accidents involving fire or heat |
| | A charged Aloe growing in your kitchen is believed to provide protection against kitchen burns and fires |
| | Burn the leaf of the aloe plant on the night of the full moon to have a new lover by the new moon |
| Aloe – Bitter | Bitter aloes powder is used to stop gossip, slander, and backbiting |
| Amber | Harmonizes the aura |
| Ambergris | Protection against evil & ill luck |
| Ambrosia | Turn a shy or timid lover into an aggressive tiger |
| | Protects from evil eye |
| Anemone | Used as a protection against sickness |
| Angelica Seed | Aids in legal matters |
| | Lengthens life and protects against disease |
| | Used to exorcise evil |
| | Protects against witchcraft, evil, spirits, spells and enchantments |

| | |
|---|---|
| Anise | Used in bath to aid clairvoyance & divination |
| | Used in purification and protection rituals |
| | Helps to keep away nightmares |
| | Used to call spirits |
| | Burn to promote prophetic dreams |
| | Burned to aid in divination |
| Apple | Attract peace of mind, contentment & happiness |
| Apple Blossom | Worn to promote happiness and success |
| | Anoint candles during love rituals |
| Apricot | Love oil to heighten passion & bind lovers together |
| Aster | Soothes ruffled feelings & calms tensions |
| Avens | Used to purify the soul |
| Azalea | Attract money & love |
| Balm | Bathe in balm to attract love |
| | Used in incense & bags to attract love |
| Balsam | Calms a person or situation |
| Bamboo | Placed over a door to ensure good luck |
| Banana | Brings victory |
| Barley | Sprinkled around the home to ward off evil |
| | Placed under door mats to repel negativity and evil |
| Basil | Relief of depression |
| | Wear to create sympathy between two people and avoid clashes |
| | Creates harmony |
| | Good for love potions, wealth, floor washes, and protection spells |
| | Rub on a green candle to attract wealth |
| | Burn as an incense to attract wealth |
| Basil – Sweet | Aids concentration |
| | Sharpens the senses |
| | Used in purification and protection rituals |
| | Draws love & prosperity |
| Bay | Aphrodisiac |
| | Stimulating & energizing |
| | Clairvoyance |
| | Psychic visions |
| | Used on the body to purify the soul |
| | Protects against evil |
| | Draws love |
| Bayberry | Anoint green candles for prosperity in the home |
| | Brings luck to the home |
| | Carry to bring money to your pocket |
| | Magnetic oil to be worn by men |
| Benzoin | Brings peace of mind |
| | Smoke is used in purification |
| Bergamot | Used in protective rituals |
| | Wear on the palm of each hand to draw prosperity |
| | Rub on money to ensure the return of riches |
| | Considered very powerful for success |
| Beth Root | Helps to attract a mate when used in a love potion |
| Betony Wood | Burn with uncrossing incense |
| | Counters hyperactivity |
| | Calms nerves |
| | Powerful against evil spirits |
| Blackberry | Used in wreaths with ivy to keep away evil spirits |
| Bistort | Carry in a yellow flannel bag to attract wealth & good fortune |

| | |
|---|---|
| Borage | Carried to generate courage and lift the spirits |
| Burdock Root | Used in purification and protection spells |
| Cayenne Pepper | Used in hexes, or to break a hex |
| | Used in love or separation spells |
| Calamus | Brings luck to the gardener |
| Carnation | Aids in psychic healing |
| Camphor | Wear to strengthen psychic powers |
| | Wear to break off with a lover and gain the ability to let go |
| Carnation | Worn to attract energy |
| Catnip | Aromatic used to attract love |
| Cedar | Attracts money |
| | Smoke is purifying |
| | Used to cure nightmares |
| | Keep cedar in your wallet or purse to attract money |
| | Aid to meditation |
| | Helps to overcome feelings of powerlessness |
| | Powerful against Witchcraft and Magic |
| Chamomile | Sleep potions |
| | Repels insects |
| | Promotes healing |
| | Attracts wealth |
| | Wash your hands with chamomile tea for good luck |
| | Use in bath or hair wash for attracting love |
| | Amulet for prosperity |
| | Protect from the evil eye |
| Cherry | Used in love & attraction magic |
| Cocoa – | Effective in love potions and spells |
| Chocolate | Aphrodisiac |
| | Mild euphoric |
| | Used to appease restless spirits |
| Cinnamon | Burned in purification incense |
| | Promotes health, vigor and libido |
| | Add to wine or food as a love |
| | Success & Prosperity |
| | Used for good luck in money matters |
| | Used for personal protection |
| | Add to incense to increase the power |
| Cinquefoil | Use as an additive in prosperity spells |
| | Brings love |
| | Aids in divination |
| | Protects from evil |
| | Hung in doorways to keep out evil spirits |
| | Used to anoint amulet and charm bags |
| Citronella | Repels Insects |
| | Attracts friends to the home |
| | Attracts customers to a place of business |
| Civit | Used in love domination |
| | Applied beneath the breasts for love drawing |
| Clove | Divination |
| | Exorcism |
| | Purification |
| | Burned to promote visions |
| | Dispels negativity |
| | Used in incense against gossip |
| | Used in incense to attract money |

|  | Used in incense to drive away negativity |
|  | Worn to attract the opposite sex |
|  | Worn to gain luck |
|  | Worn or carried to repel negative energies |
|  | Inhaled to help memory and eyesight |
| Clover | Place on lovers pillow to ensure faithfulness |
|  | Brings prosperity in business |
|  | Gives protection against evil influences |
| Coconut | Worn to ensure chastity |
|  | Anoint a fast luck candle for luck in a hurry |
| Coffee | Reverses witchcraft |
|  | Shuts down enemies |
| Coltsfoot | Added to love sachets |
|  | Used in spells for peace and tranquility |
|  | Aids in obtaining visions |
| Comfrey | Safe travel |
|  | Draws money |
|  | Protection against any type of negativity |
| Coriander | Protection of home |
|  | Used in ritual drinks, incenses for longevity and love |
|  | Powdered coriander is used as a love potion for two consenting parties |
|  | Used to anoint candles in love rituals |
| Cornflower | Promotes good eyesight |
| Cotton | Attracts good luck if thrown over the shoulder at dawn |
| Cucumber | Used to calm unruliness or ugly behavior |
| Cumin | Burned with frankincense for protection |
|  | Mix with salt and scatter to keep away evil spirits and bad luck |
|  | Steep cumin seed in wine to induce lust |
|  | Place the seeds on an object to prevent theft |
|  | Brings peace and harmony to the home when you anoint doorways with the oil once a week |
| Curry Powder | Burned to keep evil forces away |
| Cyclamen | Worn to ease childbirth |
|  | Used in love & marriage spells |
| Cypress | Brings calm, tranquility & peace of mind |
|  | Used by parents of willful children to bring them in line |
|  | Wear to screen out negative vibrations |
| Damiana | Aphrodisiac |
|  | Draws love to those who drink it as tea |
|  | Burned to enhance visions |
| Daffodil | Worn next to the heart to bring good luck |
| Dandelion | Divination |
|  | Used in a tea to enhance psychic powers |
| Devils Bane | Carry in a red flannel bag to ward of arthritis |
| Dill | Protects from evil |
|  | Seeds draw money |
|  | Flowers are used for love |
|  | Steep in hot wine for love potion |
|  | Keep in home to repel witchcraft |
|  | Hang in the doorway to protect your home |
|  | Carry to protect your person |
|  | Used in money spells |
|  | Add to a ritual bath to become irresistible to the one you desire |
| Dogwood | Rub on the outside of doorknobs so that evil will not be able to enter |
| Elder Berries | Grind & place in corners & doorway for protection & to eliminate trouble |

|  | Use the root in a tea to enhance psychic powers |
| Elecampane | Mix vervain & mistletoe to make a powerful love powder |
| Eucalyptus | Sew into a pillow to ward off nightmares |
|  | Attracts healing vibrations and protection |
|  | Cleanse any space of unwanted energies |
|  | Anoint throat, wrists & forehead for healing |
| Evergreen | Stimulates a man |
| Eyebright | Used to enhance vision |
|  | Used to enhance mental and psychic powers |
| Fennel | Place a bit of fennel in a keyhole to keep ghosts away |
|  | Used for protection spells |
|  | Prevents curses, possession and negativity |
|  | Gives strength, courage and longevity |
| Fern | Brings good luck to the person who breaks the first fern frond of Spring |
|  | Used in weather spells |
|  | Used in exorcisms |
| Feverfew | Used to ward off sickness and bolster immune system |
|  | Protects travelers |
| Fig | Divination |
|  | Fertility |
|  | Placed on the doorstep before leaving it will ensure you will arrive home safely |
| Flax Seed | Keep the peace at home |
|  | Placed in a bowl to absorb negative energy |
|  | Carry flax seeds in your wallet or purse to attract money |
| Frangipani | Love attraction oil |
|  | Causes others to tell you their secrets |
|  | Good for spiritual communications and cleansings |
|  | Used to anoint magical tools |
|  | Used in exorcisms, purification rituals, and blessings |
|  | Worn to protect against negativity |
| Galangal | Stimulating oil that helps reduce stress |
|  | Worn or carried to protect and draw good luck |
|  | Placed in a bag of leather with silver to bring money |
|  | Powdered and burned to break spells and curses |
|  | Sprinkled around the home to promote lust |
|  | Talisman to guard health |
|  | Talisman to aid psychic development |
| Gardenia | Healing |
|  | Worn to attract love |
|  | Used to bring peaceful vibrations and to attract good spirits |
|  | Protective oil worn stop others from creating strife |
|  | Cleanses aura |
|  | Brings clarity of mind |
| Geranium | Said to act as a hex breaker |
|  | Good for attraction & love |
|  | Soothing, mood-lifting, balancing |
| Ginger | Carry the root of ginger in your purse to ensure prosperity |
|  | Boil ginger root to draw power, success, and money |
|  | Used as an aphrodisiac to induce passion |
|  | Apply behind the ears to induce passion |
|  | Carry for gambling luck |
|  | Eat before performing spells to increase your power |
|  | Said to bring supernatural & magical abilities to an individual |
| Grape | Helps attract popularity |

| | |
|---|---|
| Hawthorne | Draws money |
| | Clairvoyance |
| | Divination |
| | Carry a sprig to weddings to ensure happiness for the couple |
| | Hang above a newborn's crib to provide protection |
| Hazel | Enhances mental powers |
| | Nuts are used in fertility amulets & spells |
| Heather | Anoint the purse or wallet daily to ensure you will never be without money |
| Heliotrope | Clairvoyance |
| | Protects from physical harm |
| | Attracts wealth |
| Hibiscus | Anoint the temples to draw wisdom and increase concentration |
| | Used to induce lust |
| Holly | Carried to promote good luck |
| | Hung around the house at Yule to bring good luck throughout the year |
| | Used to keep away lightning, poison, evil spirits, and negative energies |
| | The wood is used to make magical tools for use in wish magic |
| | Keeps away lightning, poison, evil spirits, and negativity |
| Holly Thistle | Sprinkle around the home to get rid of a hex |
| Honeysuckle | Dab on the temples to promote quick thinking and enhances memory |
| | Worn to increase psychic ability |
| | Used in spells to increase money |
| Hops | Used in healing incense |
| | Put inside the pillow to induce sleep |
| | Used in healing amulets |
| Horehound | Increases concentration and focus |
| | Carry or burn for protection wishes |
| | Brings blessings to the home when flowers are tied with a ribbon and hung |
| Hyacinth | Brings peace of mind to the mentally disturbed |
| | Attracts love & luck when used in the bath |
| Hyssop | Purifying baths & spells |
| | Burned as an incense to call dragon energy |
| | Aids in physical and spiritual protection |
| | Dress white candles with hyssop for uncrossing and protective spells |
| | Draws prosperity and helps to increase finances |
| Iris | Used to make the wearer attractive to others |
| Irish Moss | Carried or placed underneath rugs to increase luck & insure a steady flow of money |
| | Sprinkled around a business to bring customers |
| Iron Weed | Carry in a purple flannel bag to gain control over others |
| Jasmine | Worn to attract love |
| | Sewn into a lovers pillow so they will want only you |
| | A powerful love oil used to bind someone to you |
| | Stimulates self-confidence |
| | Used to cure insomnia & bring prophetic dreams |
| | Useful during meditation |
| Job's Tears | Three seeds are carried for good luck |
| Juniper | Used in spells for protection against evil |
| | Scent is said to aid meditation & bring spiritual enlightenment |
| | Worn to acquire wishes |
| Juniper Berries | Used as an incense for protection against magic of all kinds |
| | Burned or carried to enhance psychic powers |
| | Attracts healthy energies |
| Kava-Kava | Carry in a red flannel bag for success & promotions |
| | Protects from harm |

184

| | |
|---|---|
| | As a tea is said to induce psychic visions |
| Lavender | Aids in curing insomnia and nightmares |
| | Used in healing and purifying rituals |
| | Used to around sexual desire in men |
| | Add to wash water, burn as an incense or use in aromatics to bring happiness, love and peace to the home |
| Leather | Worn to draw friendship |
| | Helps to heal the sick when applied to the body |
| Lemon | Used by healers to aid in calling the spirits |
| | Sprayed in the home to aid in protection |
| | Leaves are used to induce lust |
| Lemon Balm | Used in healing and love spells |
| | Draws success |
| | Wear on the forehead to promote psychic powers and make contact with spirits |
| Lemongrass | Aids in using psychic powers |
| | Wear on the forehead to ease contact with spirits |
| Lilac | Induces far memory and aids in recalling past lives |
| | Induces clairvoyant powers |
| | Brings peace and harmony |
| | Worn to keep away angry spirits |
| | Anoint the back of the neck to improve the memory and draw health |
| Lily | Worn for its protective energy |
| | Used to stop manipulative love affairs |
| | Anoint the forehead to give peace and tranquility to someone who is emotionally upset |
| Lime | Helps to combat emotional apathy |
| | Attracts good fortune |
| | Used for attracting healing energies |
| | Add 3 drops to controlling incense and burn once a week to keep your mate faithful |
| Linden | Used in sleeping incense |
| | Used to increase the power of seals and talismans |
| | Added to the bathwater it helps with uncrossing |
| Lotus | Has high spiritual vibrations and is used for blessing, anointing, and meditation |
| | Wear lotus oil to receive good fortune and happiness |
| | Worn by women to draw love and incite lust |
| | Used by healers to call spirits |
| Lucky Hand | Used in sachets & bags for luck and success |
| | Carried in a red flannel bag it is said to bring luck to gamblers |
| Magnolia | Used to maintain a faithful relationship |
| | Anoint the head to aid in psychic development and obtain peace of mind |
| | Brings peace & harmony |
| Mandrake Root | Provides protection against evil |
| | Used in spells to increase psychic powers |
| | Intensifies any spell |
| | Used as a visionary herb |
| | A whole mandrake root is kept in the home to bring protection and prosperity |
| | Carried to attract love |
| | Used as a charm to promote courage |
| Marigold | Burned as a visionary herb |
| | Burn when attempting divination for love and legal matters |
| | Use in love sachets & baths to attract true love |

|  |  |
|---|---|
|  | Used to curse enemies |
| Marjoram | Used to dispel negative energy |
|  | Protects against evil |
|  | Used to induce prophetic dreams |
|  | Believed to draw love and happiness |
|  | Place in each room of the home to protect against witchcraft |
| Melon | Arouses passion, strength, energy and virility in men |
| Mimosa | Anoint the forehead before retiring to draw prophetic dreams |
| Mint | Anoint wallets or carry to draw money |
|  | Increases power of spells |
|  | Aids in ensuring save travel |
|  | Kept at a business location to draw customers |
| Mistletoe | Kept in a business to attract customers |
|  | Made into a bath for drawing love |
| Morning Glory | Carry when traveling for protection |
|  | Sprinkle about the home for protection |
|  | Place under your pillow to stop nightmares and bring beneficial dreams |
| Moss | Gravestone moss carried in the pocket ensures good luck and financial profit |
|  | Uses in witches bottles to bring prosperity to the home or business |
|  | Carry in your bra to attract the attention of a man |
| Motherwort | Keep some by the family pictures to keep them safe |
| Mustard Seed | One of the oldest good luck amulets |
| Mug wart | Hang over doorways to keep evil away |
|  | Use in spells to increase psychic powers |
|  | Use in dream pillows to draw prophetic dreams |
|  | Burn in scrying rituals |
|  | Helps to protect travelers by keeping them from getting road weary |
| Mullein | Used to keep away demons & nightmares |
|  | Protects against wild animals |
|  | Used in protection and exorcism spells |
|  | Carry to increase courage |
| Musk | Used to arouse passion and heighten sexual pleasure |
|  | Worn to increase courage |
|  | Worn to achieve success in endeavors |
|  | Use to anoint the home each morning for protection |
|  | Used in protection and hex breaking rituals |
|  | Worn as a guard against any evil direct toward the wearer |
| Myrtle | Used to quell feelings of anger |
|  | Attracts money and good fortune |
|  | Used in sleep potions |
|  | Attracts love and peace |
| Narcissus | Used in calming potions it helps to relax the mind, sooth the nerves and promote peace and harmony |
|  | Used with patchouli to create a high sexual atmosphere |
|  | Use in dream pillows to ward off nightmares and promote restful slumber |
| Neroli | Used to combat depression, anxiety, hysteria and shock |
|  | Calming |
|  | Rubbed between the breasts to attract men |
|  | Anoint the temples to bring peace |
| Nettle | Used in powders to remove curses |
|  | Sprinkle in the each room and doorway of a home to remove curses |
|  | Carry to remove a curse and send it back to the person |
| Nutmeg | Rub the oil on the third eye to help in meditation and induce sleep |
|  | Bath in nutmeg to remove a curse |
|  | Carry to draw good luck |

|  | Use in money & prosperity spells |
|---|---|
|  | To make a nutmeg amulet, drill a hole in the nut, fill the hole with quicksilver, and seal the hole with wax.  Carry in a red flannel bag for luck |
|  | Acorns are used to draw fast money |
| Olive | Leaves are worn to bring good luck |
|  | Olive is used to bring wisdom, peace and an end to arguments |
| Orange | Symbol of luck and good fortune |
|  | Added to prosperity powders, incenses and mixtures to strengthen the spell |
|  | The leaves or oils are used in love mixtures to bring on a proposal |
|  | Used to attract money and wealth |
| Orange Blossom | The oil is used to induce a marriage proposal |
|  | Women bath in it to build attractiveness in the eyes of their mate |
| Orchid | The oils are worn to attract love |
|  | Used in candle magic to inspire creativity and mental clarity |
|  | Aids in bringing clarity of mind, focus and enhancing memory |
| Orris Root | Dust on the clothes the one you want to attract their attention |
|  | Potent love oil though tot work where others have failed |
|  | Roots are hung in the house or used in a bath for protection |
| Papaya Leaves | Mix with mandrake root and burn for spell reversal |
|  | Promotes good health, friendship and comfort |
| Parsley | Promotes a long life |
|  | Carry in your shoe to make you more attractive |
|  | Use in purification and protection spells |
| Passion Flower | Bath in a tea to attract the opposite sex |
|  | Promotes emotional balance |
|  | Attracts friendship |
|  | Used in attractant prosperity spells |
|  | Used to relieve nerve pain and hysteria |
| Patchouli | Used to balance mind and overcome lethargy |
|  | Used by men to attract women |
|  | Wards off negativity and gives peace of mind |
|  | Helps to raise sexual energy |
|  | Used to increase prosperity |
| Peach | Sprinkled in the home to bring quiet and tranquility |
| Pennyroyal | Sprinkled in the home to remove a curse |
| Peony | Carry in a green bag to attract money or to attracts customers and success in business |
|  | Protects from evil spirits and storms |
|  | Used in banishing spells to rid others of negative thoughts against you |
| Peppermint | Burn before bed to induce prophetic dreams |
|  | Used in healing and purification baths |
|  | Used to create change in ones life |
| Periwinkle | Burn with love incense before having sex to bind your partner to you |
| Persimmon | Bury a green persimmon to draw good luck |
| Pine | Burn in cleansing incense to remove negativity from the home |
|  | Attracts money |
|  | Worn to cleanse the aura |
|  | Used in candle magic to draw prosperity |
|  | Bath in pine to erase past mistakes and start over |
| Pineapple | Added to baths to draw good luck to the bather |
| Plantain | Cleanses and purifies |
| Poke Root | Used in a bath to break hexes |
| Pomegranate | Used as ink in magical writings |
| Poppy Seeds | Used in dream pillows to induce slumber, calm nightmares and draw beneficial dreams |

| | |
|---|---|
| Quassia Chips | Mix with the hair of a lover and burn. Keep the ashes safe to preserve the love |
| Queen of the Meadow | Used as a tea to draw good luck |
| Raspberry Leaf | Promotes sleep |
| | Induces visions |
| Rattlesnake Root | Carry in a purple flannel bag for protection from harm |
| Rose | Added to baths to induce peace and harmony |
| | Used to promote thoughts of love |
| Rose Geranium | Anoint openings of a house for protection |
| | Worn to draw courage |
| Rosehips | Used to increase psychic power |
| | Divination |
| Rosemary | Increases memory |
| | Burn to purify and cleanse a space |
| | Protects against evil & negativity |
| | Used with juniper to purify the air |
| | Drop rosemary in coffins to reassure the dead that you won't forget them |
| | Used as protection against physical injury |
| | Believed to help special enterprises succeed |
| | Anoint the temples to aid mental powers, ease pain & promote healing |
| | Used to promote common sense and confidence |
| | Used to inspire loyalty & devotion |
| Rue | Bath in rue to attract love |
| | Carry rue in a red bag for protection |
| Saffron | Wear to aid in the development of clairvoyant powers |
| | Used to promote long life |
| Sage | Kept alive in a business, the business will thrive as the plant thrives |
| | Used to ward off misfortune |
| | Added to purification washes for the home and the self |
| | Draws healing, prosperity and wisdom |
| Sandalwood | Used for love, health and fortune |
| | Believed to grant wishes |
| | Known to be one of the most spiritual oils |
| | Protective |
| | Healing |
| | Aids one in seeing past incantations |
| | Anoint the forehead to promote sight |
| Sarsaparilla | Believed to prolong life |
| | Carried in the wallet it helps money go further |
| | Sprinkle in court to obtain a favorable decision |
| | Used in spells to obtain money |
| Sesame | Used in healing rituals to give hope to one who is sick |
| Smartweed | Attracts money |
| | Used to clear the mind |
| Snake Root | Rub on the palms to dominate an individual |
| Solomon's Seal | The roots are used to scare off evil |
| | The flowers are used in love potions |
| | Believed to heal wounds and broken bones |
| Southernwood | Burned as an incense to protect one from trouble |
| | Kept in the home as a love charm |
| Spearmint | Kept in the home to protect from attack, danger and intruders |
| Spikenard | Used to keep a mate from straying |
| St John's Root | Hang above doors and windows to protect the home from evil & witchcraft |
| | Burn to banish negative thoughts and energies |

| | |
|---|---|
| | Carry to strengthen courage |
| Straw | Used in bags to draw luck |
| | Kept in the home to draw luck |
| | Sew straw and a small horseshoe in a small bag and place it above the bed to draw luck to the sleeping person |
| Strawberry | Attractant oil for good fortune money, & love |
| Sumbul Root | Carry on you to attract love quickly |
| Sweet grass | Powerful cleanser and protector |
| | Hang a braid of sweet grass over the door to keep positive energies flowing |
| | Used to soften sad memories and allow one to move on |
| Sweet Pea | Worn on the wrists, forearms and back of the knees to attract friends and lovers |
| | Draws love and money |
| Tarragon | Dispels apathy and boredom |
| Thistle | Used to bring financial blessings |
| | Amulet for joy, energy, and vitality |
| | Burn as an incense for protection and to remove a course |
| Thyme | Used to inspire courage |
| | Used to draw the spirits of loved ones close |
| | Used in a bath to ensure money is always available |
| | Keep in a jar in the home to draw good luck |
| | Place in pillows to stop nightmares |
| | Worn to increase psychic powers |
| | Burn for purification and protection from negativity |
| Tonka | Used in love and prosperity spells |
| Tuberose | Use in a bath to draw fast luck |
| | Promotes peace & aids psychic powers |
| | Worn by men to attract women |
| Valerian | Used to cure insomnia, anxiety and tension |
| | Sprinkle in the home to end strife |
| | Added to incense this helps to get fighting couples together and restore peace, harmony and togetherness |
| | A live valerian plant in the home will help keep balance and harmony |
| Vanilla | Used as an energy restorer |
| | Used to promote extra power in magical ceremonies |
| | Increases lustful and loving energies |
| Verbena | Used in the bath to aid in learning faster |
| | Burn to help remove a curse |
| Vervain | Aids those in the performing and creative arts & stimulates creativity |
| | Used in obtaining material objects |
| | Aids in visionary work |
| | Promotes love, lust, and sexual attraction |
| | Helps to reconcile enemies |
| Vetiver | Placed in cash registers to increase business |
| | Carried to attract luck |
| | Burn to overcome evil spells |
| Violet | Carry to bring changes in luck or fortune |
| | Used with other attraction herbs in drawing spells |
| | Oils are used to attract a lover and to bring peace and marital happiness |
| | Used in candle magic to repel negativity |
| | Used to overcome any spell cast against you |
| White Willow | Carry to attract love |
| | Used in healing spells |
| | Burn to conjure spirits |

| | |
|---|---|
| Wisteria | Believed to open the doorway between man and god it is used as a path to higher consciousness & illumination |
| | Add to house washes to attract good fortune & prosperity |
| Wood Rose | Carried to attract good luck and fortune |
| | Placed in the home to draw luck |
| Yarrow | To overcome fear, carry in a yellow flannel bag with a parchment detailing your fears |
| | Carry to repel negative influences |
| | Use to keep a happy marriage |
| Ylang-Ylang | Used to attract love, money, & opportunity |
| | used to make wearer irresistible |
| | Used to sooth problems in married life |
| | Helps calm during interviews |

# HERB CORRESPONDENCES BY GOAL

Luck

Allspice Berries
Good luck charms
Aloe Hung over houses and doors to bring good luck
Ambergris Protection against evil & ill luck
Bamboo Placed over a door to ensure good luck
Bayberry Brings luck to the home
Bistort Carry in a yellow flannel bag to attract wealth & good fortune
Calamus Brings luck to the gardener
Chamomile Wash your hands with chamomile tea for good luck
Clove Worn to gain luck
Coconut Anoint a fast luck candle for luck in a hurry
Cotton Attracts good luck if thrown over the shoulder at dawn
Daffodil Worn next to the heart to bring good luck
Galangal Worn or carried to protect and draw good luck
Ginger Carry for gambling luck
Holly Carried to promote good luck
Holly Hung around the house at Yule to bring good luck throughout the year
Job's Tears Three seeds are carried for good luck
Lotus Wear lotus oil to receive good fortune and happiness
Lucky Hand Used in sachets & bags for luck and success
Lucky Hand Carried in a red flannel bag it is said to bring luck to gamblers
Mustard Seed One of the oldest good luck amulets
Myrtle Attracts money and good fortune
Nutmeg Carry to draw good luck To make a nutmeg amulet, drill a hole in the nut, fill the hole with quicksilver and seal the hole with wax
Nutmeg Carry in a red flannel bag for luck
Olive Leaves are worn to bring good luck
Orange Symbol of luck and good fortune
Persimmon Bury a green persimmon to draw good luck
Pineapple Added to baths to draw good luck to the bather
Queen of the Meadow Used as a tea to draw good luck
Straw Used in bags to draw luck
Straw Kept in the home to draw luck
Straw Sew straw and a small horseshoe in a small bag and place it above the bed to draw luck to the sleeping person
Thyme Keep in a jar in the home to draw good luck
Tuberose Use in a bath to draw fast luck
Vetiver Carried to attract luck
Violet Carry to bring changes in luck or fortune
Wisteria Add to house washes to attract good fortune & prosperity
Wood Rose Carried to attract good luck and fortune
Wood Rose Placed in the home to draw luck

Legal

Angelica Seed Aids in legal matters
Banana Brings victory
Sarsaparilla Sprinkle in court to obtain a favorable decision

| Prosperity | |
|---|---|
| | Allspice Brings prosperity, health & protection |
| | Almond Attract money, good fortune & wealth |
| | Almond Added to money incenses & potions |
| | Alfalfa Brings good fortune in matters of money, business and good luck in gambling |
| | Alfalfa Keep sprigs in the home or as part of a mojo bag to keep poverty away & help you prosper |
| | All Spice Burned as an incense to attract money or luck |
| | Allspice Berries Draws fortune in business and gambling |
| | Almond Used to anoint money & candles in prosperity rituals |
| | Almond Used in money incense |
| | Azalea Attract money & love |
| | Basil Rub on a green candle to attract wealth |
| | Basil Burn as an incense to attract wealth |
| | Basil – Sweet Draws love & prosperity |
| | Bayberry Anoint green candles for prosperity in the home |
| | Bayberry Carry to bring money to your pocket |
| | Bergamot Wear on the palm of each hand to draw prosperity |
| | Bergamot Rub on money to ensure the return of riches |
| | Bistort Carry in a yellow flannel bag to attract wealth & good fortune |
| | Cedar Attracts money |
| | Cedar Keep cedar in your wallet or purse to attract money |
| | Chamomile Attracts wealth |
| | Chamomile Amulet for prosperity |
| | Cinnamon Success & Prosperity |
| | Cinnamon Used for good luck in money matters |
| | Cinquefoil Use as an additive in prosperity spells |
| | Clove Used in incense to attract money |
| | Comfrey Draws money |
| | Dill Seeds draw money |
| | Dill Used in money spells |
| | Flax Seed Carry flax seeds in your wallet or purse to attract money |
| | Galangal Placed in a bag of leather with silver to bring money |
| | Ginger Carry the root of ginger in your purse to ensure prosperity |
| | Ginger Boil ginger root to draw power, success, and money |
| | Grape Draws money |
| | Heather Anoint the purse or wallet daily to ensure you will never be without money |
| | Heliotrope Attracts wealth |
| | Honeysuckle Used in spells to increase money |
| | Hyssop Draws prosperity and helps to increase finances |
| | Irish Moss Carried or placed underneath rugs to increase luck & insure a steady flow of money |
| | Lime Attracts good fortune |
| | Mandrake Root A whole mandrake root is kept in the home to bring |
| | Mint Anoint wallets or carry to draw money |
| | Moss Gravestone moss carried in the pocket ensures good luck and financial profit |
| | Moss Uses in witches bottles to bring prosperity to the home or business |
| | Myrtle Attracts money and good fortune |
| | Nutmeg Use in money & prosperity spells |
| | Acorns are used to draw fast money |
| | Orange Added to prosperity powders, incenses and mixtures to strengthen the spell |

192

Orange Used to attract money and wealth
Passion Flower Used in attractant prosperity spells
Patchouli Used to increase prosperity
Peony Carry in a green bag to attract money
Pine Attracts money
Pine Used in candle magic to draw prosperity
Sage Draws prosperity
Sarsaparilla Carried in the wallet it helps money go further
Sarsaparilla Used in spells to obtain money
Smartweed Attracts money
Strawberry Attractant oil for good fortune money, & love
Sweet Pea Draws love and money
Thistle Used to bring financial blessings
Thyme Used in a bath to ensure money is always available
Thyme Used to attract money & opportunity

**Cleansing**

Angelica Seed Used to exorcise evil
Anise Used in purification and protection rituals
Basil – Sweet Used in purification and protection rituals
Burdock Root Used in purification and protection spells
Cinnamon Burned in purification incense
Eucalyptus Cleanse any space of unwanted energies
Frangipani Used in exorcisms, purification rituals, and blessings
Hyssop Purifying baths & spells
Marjoram Used to dispel negative energy
Pine Burn in cleansing incense to remove negativity from the home
Rosemary Burn to purify and cleanse a space
Rosemary Used with juniper to purify the air
Sage Added to purification washes for the home and the self
St John's Root Burn to banish negative thoughts and energies
Sweet grass Powerful cleanser and protector
Thyme Burn for purification and protection from negativity

**Courage**

Borage Carried to generate courage and lift the spirits
Cedar Helps to overcome feelings of powerlessness
Fennel Gives strength, courage
Mandrake Root Used as a charm to promote courage
Mullein Carry to increase courage
Musk Worn to increase courage
Rose Geranium Worn to draw courage
St John's Root Carry to strengthen courage
Thyme Used to inspire courage
Yarrow To overcome fear, carry in a yellow flannel bag with a parchment detailing your fears

**Nasty People**

Aloe – Bitter powder is used to stop gossip, slander, and backbiting
Clove Used in incense against gossip
Cucumber Used to calm unruliness or ugly behavior
Gardenia Protective oil worn stop others from creating strife
Iron Weed Carry in a purple flannel bag to gain control over others

| House Protection | Elder Berries Grind & place in corners & doorway for protection & to eliminate trouble |
| --- | --- |
| | Barley Sprinkled around the home to ward off evil |
| | Barley Placed under door mats to repel negativity and evil |
| | Blackberry Used in wreaths with ivy to keep away evil spirits |
| | Cinquefoil Hung in doorways to keep out evil spirits |
| | Clove Used in incense to drive away negativity |
| | Comfrey Protection against any type of negativity |
| | Coriander Protection of home |
| | Cumin Mix with salt and scatter to keep away evil spirits and bad luck |
| | Cumin Brings peace and harmony to the home when you anoint doorways with the oil once a week |
| | Curry Powder Burned to keep evil forces away |
| | Dill Keep in home to repel witchcraft |
| | Dill Hang in the doorway to protect your home |
| | Dogwood Rub on the outside of doorknobs so that evil will not be able to enter |
| | Flax Seed Placed in a bowl to absorb negative energy |
| | Juniper Berries Used as an incense for protection against magic of all kinds |
| | Lemon Sprayed in the home to aid in protection |
| | Mandrake Root A whole mandrake root is kept in the home to bring protection |
| | Marjoram Place in each room of the home to protect against witchcraft |
| | Morning Glory Sprinkle about the home for protection |
| | Mug wart Hang over doorways to keep evil away |
| | Musk Use to anoint the home each morning for protection |
| | Orris Root Roots are hung in the house or used in a bath for protection |
| | Patchouli Wards off negativity and gives peace of mind |
| | Rose Geranium Anoint openings of a house for protection |
| | Spearmint Kept in the home to protect from attack, danger and intruders |
| | St John's Root Hang above doors and windows to protect the home from evil & witchcraft |
| | Sweet grass Hang a braid of sweet grass over the door to keep positive energies flowing |
| | Thistle Burn as an incense for protection and to remove a curse |
| | |
| Personal Protection | Chamomile Protect from the evil eye |
| | Cinnamon Used for personal protection |
| | Clove Worn or carried to repel negative energies |
| | Clover Gives protection against evil influences |
| | Comfrey Protection against any type of negativity |
| | Cypress Wear to screen out negative vibrations |
| | Dill Carry to protect your person |
| | Frangipani Worn to protect against negativity |
| | Heliotrope Protects from physical harm |
| | Hyssop Aids in physical and spiritual protection |
| | Lilac Worn to keep away angry spirits |
| | Lily Worn for its protective energy |
| | Musk Worn as a guard against any evil direct toward the wearer |
| | Rattlesnake Root Carry in a purple flannel bag for protection from harm |
| | Rosemary Used as protection against physical injury |
| | Rue Carry rue in a red bag for protection |
| | Yarrow Carry to repel negative influences |

| Hexes / Curses | Agrimony Burn to reverse & turn back spells |
| | Ague Weed Burn to stop hexes & crossings from getting to you |
| | Betony Wood Burn with uncrossing incense |
| | Cayenne Pepper Used in hexes, or to break a hex |
| | Coffee Reverses witchcraft |
| | Coffee Shuts down enemies |
| | Galangal Powdered and burned to break spells and curses |
| | Geranium Said to act as a hex breaker |
| | Holly Thistle Sprinkle around the home to get rid of a hex |
| | Hyssop Dress white candles with hyssop for uncrossing and protective spells |
| | Linden Added to the bathwater it helps with uncrossing |
| | Musk Used in protection and hex breaking rituals |
| | Nettle Used in powders to remove curses |
| | Nettle Sprinkle in the each room and doorway of a home to remove curses |
| | Nettle Carry to remove a curse and send it back to the person |
| | Nutmeg Bath in nutmeg to remove a curse |
| | Pennyroyal Sprinkled in the home to remove a curse |
| | Verbena Burn to help remove a curse |
| | Vetiver Burn to overcome evil spells |
| | Violet Used to overcome any spell cast against you |

| Success-Confidence | Apple Blossom Worn to promote happiness and success |
| | Bergamot Considered very powerful for success |
| | Jasmine Stimulates self-confidence |
| | Kava-Kava Carry in a red flannel bag for success & promotions |
| | Lemon Balm Draws success |
| | Musk Worn to achieve success in endeavors |
| | Rosemary Believed to help special enterprises succeed & promote confidence |

| Fighting | Aster Soothes ruffled feelings & calms tensions |
| | Balsam Calms a person or situation |
| | Basil Wear to create sympathy between two people and avoid clashes |
| | Basil Creates harmony |
| | Coltsfoot Used in spells for peace and tranquility |
| | Cucumber Used to calm unruliness or ugly behavior |
| | Cypress Used by parents of willful children to bring them in line |
| | Flax Seed Keep the peace at home |
| | Gardenia Protective oil worn stop others from creating strife |
| | Lavender Add to wash water, burn as an incense or use in aromatics to bring happiness, love and peace to the home |
| | Iron Weed Carry in a purple flannel bag to gain control over others |
| | Lilac Brings peace and harmony |
| | Olive Olive is used to bring wisdom, peace and an end to arguments |
| | Peach Sprinkled in the home to bring quiet and tranquility |
| | Valerian Sprinkle in the home to end strife |
| | Valerian Added to incense this helps to get fighting couples together and restore peace, harmony and togetherness |
| | Valerian A live valerian plant in the home will help keep balance and harmony |

| | |
|---|---|
| Business | Citronella Attracts customers to a place of business |
| | Clover Brings prosperity in business |
| | Irish Moss Sprinkled around a business to bring customers |
| | Mint Kept at a business location to draw customers |
| | Mistletoe Kept in a business to attract customers |
| | Peony Carry in a green bag to attracts customers and success in business |
| | Sage Kept alive in a business, the business will thrive as the plant thrives |
| | Vetiver Placed in cash registers to increase business |
| | |
| Travel | Comfrey Safe travel |
| | Feverfew Protects travelers |
| | Mint Aids in ensuring save travel |
| | Morning Glory Carry when traveling for protection |
| | Mug wart Helps to protect travelers by keeping them from getting road weary |
| | |
| Wish | Horehound Carry or burn for protection wishes |
| | Juniper Worn to acquire wishes |
| | Sandalwood Believed to grant wishes |
| | Vervain Used in obtaining material objects |
| | |
| Friendship | Citronella Attracts friends to the home |
| | Grape Helps attract popularity |
| | Iris Used to make the wearer attractive to others |
| | Leather Worn to draw friendship |
| | Passion Flower Attracts friendship |
| | Sweet Pea Worn on the wrists, forearms and back of the knees to attract friends |
| | |
| Love For Men | Bayberry Magnetic oil to be worn by men |
| | Patchouli Used by men to attract women |
| | Tuberose Worn by men to attract women |
| | |
| Love For Women | Evergreen Stimulates a man |
| | Lavender Used to arouse sexual desire in men |
| | Lotus Worn by women to draw love and incite lust |
| | Neroli Rubbed between the breasts to attract men |
| | Orange Blossom Women bath in it to build attractiveness in the eyes of their mate |
| | Melon Arouses passion, strength, energy and virility in men |

New Love

Aloe Burn the leaf of the aloe plant on the night of the full moon to have a new lover by the new moon
Azalea Attract love
Balm Bathe in balm to attract love
Balm Used in incense & bags to attract love
Basil – Sweet Draws love
Bay Draws love
Beth Root Helps to attract a mate when used in a love potion
Catnip Aromatic used to attract love
Chamomile Use in bath or hair wash for attracting love
Cherry Used in love & attraction magic
Cinnamon Add to wine or food as a love
Cinquefoil Brings love
Civit Applied beneath the breasts for love drawing
Civit Used in love domination
Clove Worn to attract the opposite sex
Coltsfoot Added to love sachets
Coriander Used to anoint candles in love rituals
Damiana Draws love to those who drink it as tea
Dill Flowers are used for love
Dill Add to a ritual bath to become irresistible to the one you desire
Frangipani Love attraction oil
Gardenia Worn to attract love
Geranium Good for attraction & love
Hyacinth Attracts love & luck when used in the bath
Jasmine Worn to attract love
Mandrake Root Carried to attract love
Marigold Use in love sachets & baths to attract true love
Marjoram Believed to draw love and happiness
Mistletoe Made into a bath for drawing love
Moss Carry in your bra to attract the attention of a man
Myrtle Attracts love
Orchid The oils are worn to attract love
Parsley Carry in your shoe to make you more attractive
Passion Flower Bath in a tea to attract the opposite sex
Rose Used to promote thoughts of love
Rue Bath in rue to attract love
Solomon's Seal The flowers are used in love potions
Sumbul Root Carry on you to attract love quickly
Sweet Pea Worn on the wrists, forearms and back of the knees to attract friends and lovers
Vervain Promotes love, lust, and sexual attraction
White Willow Carry to attract love
Ylang-Ylang Used to attract love
Ylang-Ylang Used to make wearer irresistible
Apple Blossom Anoint candles during love rituals

| Strengthen Love | Ambrosia Turn a shy or timid lover into an aggressive tiger |
|---|---|
| | Apricot Love oil to heighten passion & bind lovers together |
| | Bay Aphrodisiac |
| | Coriander Used to anoint candles in love rituals |
| | Cyclamen Used in love & marriage spells |
| | Damiana Aphrodisiac |
| | Dill Add to a ritual bath to become irresistible to the one you desire |
| | Galangal Sprinkled around the home to promote lust |
| | Ginger Apply behind the ears to induce passion |
| | Hibiscus Used to induce lust |
| | Jasmine Sewn into a lovers pillow so they will want only you |
| | Jasmine A powerful love oil used to bind someone to you |
| | Lavender Add to wash water, burn as an incense or use in aromatics to bring happiness, love and peace to the home |
| | Lemon Leaves are used to induce lust |
| | Lime Add 3 drops to controlling incense and burn once a week to keep your mate faithful |
| | Magnolia Used to maintain a faithful relationship |
| | Musk Used to arouse passion and heighten sexual pleasure |
| | Narcissus Used with patchouli to create a high sexual atmosphere |
| | Orange The leaves or oils are used in love mixtures to bring on a proposal |
| | Orange Blossom The oil is used to induce a marriage proposal |
| | Patchouli Helps to raise sexual energy |
| | Periwinkle Burn with love incense before having sex to bind your partner to you |
| | Southernwood Kept in the home as a love charm |
| | Spikenard Used to keep a mate from straying |
| | Vanilla Increases lustful and loving energies |
| | Violet Oils are used to attract a lover and to bring peace and marital happiness |
| | Yarrow Use to keep a happy marriage |
| | Ylang-Ylang Used to sooth problems in married life |
| | Clover Place on lovers pillow to ensure faithfulness |
| | Apple Blossom Anoint candles during love rituals |
| | |
| Separate – Get Over Love | Cayenne Pepper Used in love or separation spells |
| | |
| | Camphor Wear to break off with a lover and gain the ability to let go |
| | |
| | Lily Used to stop manipulative love affairs |
| | |
| Meditation | Acacia - Worn to aid meditation |
| | Acacia Divination |
| | Cedar Aid to meditation |
| | Jasmine Useful during meditation |
| | Juniper Scent is said to aid meditation & bring spiritual enlightenment |
| | Lotus Has high spiritual vibrations and is used meditation |
| | Nutmeg Rub the oil on the third eye to help in meditation |

| | |
|---|---|
| Divination | Anise Used in bath to aid clairvoyance & divination |
| | Anise Burn to promote prophetic dreams |
| | Anise Burned to aid in divination |
| | Bay Clairvoyance |
| | Cinquefoil Aids in divination |
| | Clove Divination |
| | Dandelion Divination |
| | Hawthorne Clairvoyance |
| | Hawthorne Divination |
| | Lilac Induces clairvoyant powers |
| | Saffron Wear to aid in the development of clairvoyant powers |
| | |
| Prophetic Dreams | Jasmine Used to cure insomnia & bring prophetic dreams |
| | Marjoram Used to induce prophetic dreams |
| | Mug wart Use in dream pillows to draw prophetic dreams |
| | Peppermint Burn before bed to induce prophetic dreams |
| | Mimosa Anoint the forehead before retiring to draw prophetic dreams |
| | |
| Past Lives | Lilac Induces far memory and aids in recalling past lives |
| | Sandalwood Aids one in seeing past incantations |
| | |
| Visions | Bay Psychic visions |
| | Coltsfoot Aids in obtaining visions |
| | Damiana Burned to enhance visions |
| | Eyebright Used to enhance vision |
| | Kava-Kava As a tea is said to induce psychic visions |
| | Mandrake Root Used as a visionary herb |
| | Marigold Burned as a visionary herb |
| | Raspberry Leaf Induces visions |
| | Wisteria Believed to open the doorway between man and god it is used as a path to higher consciousness & illumination |
| | Clove Burned to promote visions |
| | |
| Increase Power | Acacia Develop psychic powers |
| | Camphor Wear to strengthen psychic powers |
| | Dandelion Used in a tea to enhance psychic powers |
| | Elder Berries Use the root in a tea to enhance psychic powers |
| | Eyebright Used to enhance mental and psychic powers |
| | Galangal Talisman to aid psychic development |
| | Ginger Eat before performing spells to increase your power |
| | Ginger Said to bring supernatural & magical abilities to an individual |
| | Hazel Enhances mental powers |
| | Honeysuckle Worn to increase psychic ability |
| | Juniper Berries Burned or carried to enhance psychic powers |
| | Lemongrass Aids in using psychic powers |
| | Magnolia Anoint the head to aid in psychic development |
| | Mandrake Root Used in spells to increase psychic powers |
| | Mug wart Use in spells to increase psychic powers |
| | Rosehips Used to increase psychic power |
| | Thyme Worn to increase psychic powers |
| | Tuberose Promotes peace & aids psychic powers |

Spirits

Frangipani Good for spiritual communications and cleansings
Lemongrass Wear on the forehead to ease contact with spirits
White Willow Burn to conjure spirits
Anise Used to call spirits
Thyme Used to draw the spirits of loved ones close

# *Timing*

Some people believe that that the phase of the moon, day of the week, or month of the year affect the ability of a particular practice to succeed. While you can complete a ritual or spell at any time of the day or night or season of the year and achieve the results you desire, you may want to consider the correspondences commonly believed to affect the energies of the world around you.

# *Moon Correspondences*

Waxing Moon      It is often beneficial to complete spells involving growth healing, initiation of something new, love, luck, sex, and positive magic during the waxing moon

Full Moon      It is often beneficial to complete spells involving completion, dreams, fertility, psychic ability, and spiritual enlightenment during the full moon

Waning Moon      The waning moon is the time that many people complete banishment and reversal spells to remove obstacles, neutralize enemies, and remove harm

New Moon  This is the time to work spells for growth and new beginnings with the understanding that the benefits may not manifest until after the appearance of the full moon

## *Creating Your Own Spells*

You know have a beginner's understanding of the fundamentals of spell craft, the uses of various components in spell work, and the processes that might be employed to channel the energies of the world around you.

There are many guides that detail exact spells created by others just as if this guide gives you a few starter spells that you can use. These will likely work well enough for simple tasks but the most powerful effects will come from those spells, formulas, and rituals you design for yourself.

Each of us holds energies that can be properly channeled and focused to create the effects we desire. Many people find that it is easiest to access these energies when we have a guide and tangible tools to use as a starting point. You know have your starting point. If you have moved through this guide to reach these final pages, you are ready to expand your horizons and branch into creation of your own.

Always remember to ground, center, and shield yourself before beginning any ritual. Your tools and components must always be fully cleansed and charged.

Blessings on your journey.

# Locator Guide

www.ingramcontent.com/pod-product-compliance
Lightning Source LLC
Chambersburg PA
CBHW081823280526
45789CB00007B/2318